1 MONTH OF FREE READING

at

www.ForgottenBooks.com

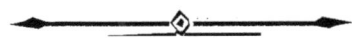

By purchasing this book you are eligible for one month membership to ForgottenBooks.com, giving you unlimited access to our entire collection of over 1,000,000 titles via our web site and mobile apps.

To claim your free month visit: www.forgottenbooks.com/free783015

* Offer is valid for 45 days from date of purchase. Terms and conditions apply.

ISBN 978-0-260-95558-6
PIBN 10783015

This book is a reproduction of an important historical work. Forgotten Books uses state-of-the-art technology to digitally reconstruct the work, preserving the original format whilst repairing imperfections present in the aged copy. In rare cases, an imperfection in the original, such as a blemish or missing page, may be replicated in our edition. We do, however, repair the vast majority of imperfections successfully; any imperfections that remain are intentionally left to preserve the state of such historical works.

Forgotten Books is a registered trademark of FB &c Ltd.
Copyright © 2018 FB &c Ltd.
FB &c Ltd, Dalton House, 60 Windsor Avenue, London, SW19 2RR.
Company number 08720141. Registered in England and Wales.

For support please visit www.forgottenbooks.com

SEMI-CENTENNIAL CELEBRATION

—OF THE—

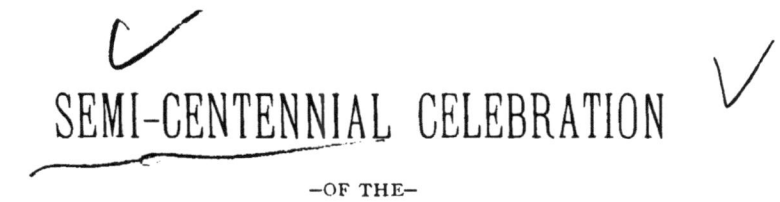

INTRODUCTION * OF * HOMŒOPATHY

WEST OF THE ALLEGHENY MOUNTAINS,

—HELD AT—

PITTSBURGH, PENN'A,

September 20th, 1887,

Under the auspices of the Homœopathic Medical Society of Allegheny County, Pa.

PUBLISHED BY THE SOCIETY.

EDITED BY J. C. BURGHER, M.D.

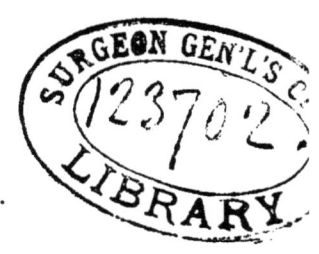

PITTSBURGH:
From the Press of Stevenson & Foster, 529 Wood Street.
1888.

WBK
H765s
1888

Film 7555, Item 4

Semi-Centennial Celebration.

Committee of Arrangements

Appointed by the Homœopathic Medical Society of Allegheny County, Penn'a.

J. H. McCLELLAND, M D.,
L. H. WILLARD, M.D.,
J. C. BURGHER, M.D.

PROGRAMME

OF THE

CELEBRATION OF THE FIFTIETH ANNIVERSARY

OF THE

INTRODUCTION OF HOMŒOPATHY

WEST OF THE ALLEGHENIES,

IN THE PERSON OF

GUSTAVUS REICHHELM, M. D.

GRAND OPERA HOUSE, PITTSBURGH,

SEPT. 20, 1887, 3: P. M.

OVERTURE—*Martha*,	Toerge's Orchestra.
INVOCATION,	By Rev. Samuel Maxwell, Pittsburgh, Pa.
HISTORIC ADDRESS,	By J. P. Dake, M. D., Nashville, Tenn.
MUSIC—IDYL—*The Shepherd Boy*,	Toerge's Orchestra.
ADDRESS,	By A. R. Thomas, M. D., Philadelphia, Pa.
MUSIC—L'ESPRIT—*Française*,	Toerge's Orchestra.
ADDRESS,	By. J. C. Burgher, M. D., Pittsburgh, Pa.
MUSIC—*Treasure from Gypsy Baron*,	Toerge's Orchestra.
ADDRESS,	By D. S. Smith, M. D., Chicago, Ill.
MUSIC—GAVOTTE—*Solitude*,	Toerge's Orchestra.
ADDRESS,	By J. W. Dowling, M. D., New York.
MUSIC—VALSE,	Toerge's Orchestra.
POEM—"*Dogmatic Doctors*,"	By Wm. Tod Helmuth, M. D., N. Y.
MUSIC—MARCH—*Silver Lake*,	Toerge's Orchestra.

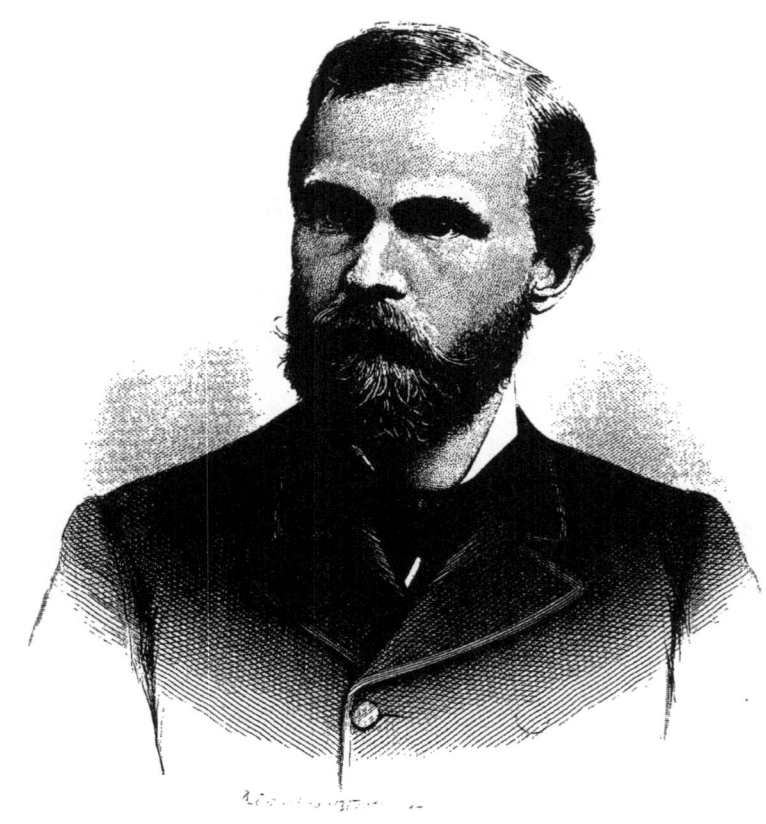

Semi-Centennial Celebration.

The celebration of the Fiftieth Anniversary of the Crossing of Homœopathy West of the Alleghenies, in the person of Gustavus Reichhelm, M.D., was held in the "Grand Opera House," Fifth Avenue, Pittsburgh, Pa., at 3.00 o'clock, P. M., Tuesday, September 20th, 1887. Some one hundred prominent Homœopathic physicians from different parts of the State and several from other States were present, the chairs and private boxes were filled by a select audience in response to special invitations issued by the Committee of Arrangements.

Toerge's Celebrated Orchestra furnished suitable music for the occasion.

J. H. McClelland, M.D., Director of ceremonies, called the assembly to order, and requested the Rev. Samuel Maxwell, Rector of Trinity Episcopal Church, to open the exercises with prayer, after which he introduced to the audience J. P. Dake, M.D., of Nashville, Tenn., as the historian of the occasion.

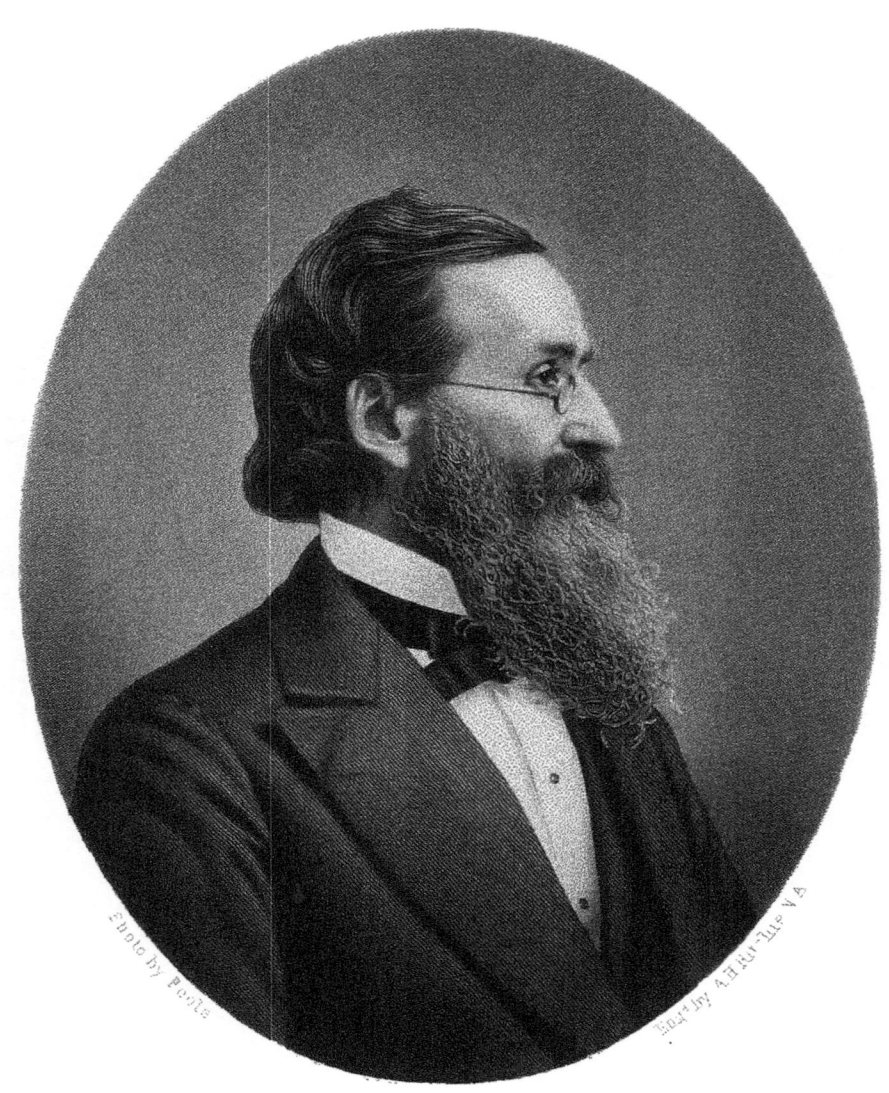

The Passage of Homoeopathy West of the Alleghenies.

An Address Delivered at the Opening of the Celebration of the Fiftieth Anniversary of the Passage of Homœopathy West of the Allegheny Mountains, Pittsburgh, Pa., Sept. 20th, 1887.

By Jabez P. Dake, A.M., M.D., Nashville, Tenn.

Mr. President, Ladies and Gentlemen:

In the course of time there come anniversary days and seasons to mark the lapse of years and the progress gained from the birth of honored leaders, the founding of cherished institutions, and the announcement of new ideas, destined to work great changes in the conditions of men.

We are assembled, to-day, to celebrate the fiftieth year since the passage of a new and most beneficent mode of healing west of the Allegheny Mountains.

The sound of the voice of the orator, the booming of cannon, and the strains of pleasing music are just dying away at the other extremity of this great commonwealth, brought forth in commemoration of the adoption of the Constitution of the American Republic just one hundred years ago.

On this ground, where we are now assembled, we might celebrate the displacement of savage rule by the coming of the French and the planting of Fort Duquesne at the confluence of the Allegheny and Monongahela rivers. And, later, we might gladly celebrate the establishment and extension of Anglo-Saxon civilization from this point.

It was here that our young Washington came when it was necessary to gain a position commanding the great territory west of the Alleghenies.

While the extension of civilization, the triumph of arms taken up in a good cause, and the adoption of a constitution, rightly termed the *maxima carta* of a free people, are events always worthy of commemoration, we hold that a move that leads to the banishment from the practice of the healing art of measures in the main useless and injurious, cruel and revolting, and the introduction of those that are more curative, while in every way agreeable, is an event calling for a joyful remembrance by all the people.

The fruits of conquest, the possession of country, home and kindred are of little worth to those who are prostrated by disease and racked with pain, in the absence of some efficient ministry of cure to bring relief.

Scarcely a single decade had gone by since the advent of Homœopathy in America, and it was practically known only in a few of the cities on the Atlantic sea-board, when a call came to the little band of medical reformers, at work in and near the city of Philadelphia, for a disciple of Hahnemann to be sent to the relief of the sick and drug-burdened people of Pittsburgh.

THE FIRST CALL.

Rev. Father Byer, a Catholic clergyman, stationed in this city, having witnessed among the sick and, doubtless, experienced in his own person, the advantages of the new mode of healing, wrote a letter to Dr. Constantine Hering, asking for one of its practitioners. The request was laid before some of the younger men, who had been in attendance at the first post-graduate medical school planted in America, the Allentown Academy of Homœopathy.

Among those asked to consider the call to Pittsburgh, was a young Prussian, educated at the University of Halle, and made acquainted with the new therapeutic principles by Wesselhœft, Hering and others of the Allentown faculty. After a brief pause he decided to accept the call.

That educated and elegant physician, destined to be the pioneer of the new therapeutics in the grand empire of states lying west of the Alleghenies was *Gustavus Reichhelm*.

THE PIONEER.

Early in the autumn of 1837 he was slowly making his way over the mountains westward.

On a bright October day, when the fields of living green were becoming bronzed, and the woodland decorated with tints of purple and gold, he approached the scene of his future toil and combat with medical ignorance and opposition as well as with human ailments.

As the softening haze on hill side and valley, peculiar to the season, hid from view the rugged and forbidding features of the distant landscape and cast a charm over all, so did the influences of youthful vigor and buoyancy, and the enthusiasm of a free and expanded son of the old Fatherland hide from anticipation all thought of the frowning prejudice and many annoyances that were awaiting him. Gladly received by Father Byer and a few others, who had been induced to seek relief and length of days by the novel method, Reichhelm began his work here on the 10th day of October, 1837. Known at first, as the "Dutch Doctor," and then the "Sugar-powder Doctor," he moved quietly on, provoking only smiles of derision from the medical men around him. He was employed as attending physician at the Catholic Orphan Asylum, where the cures effected attracted much attention and inspired confidence in the new practice.

During a period of nearly twelve years, under his medical administration, and with several epidemics of measles, whooping-cough and scarlet fever, there were but two deaths among the inmates of the institution. And it should be remarked that one of the fatal cases was that of a child, taken from a mother prostrated with consumption, itself dying from inanition a few days after admission.

I had a statement from one of the old visitors of the Asylum, that more children died during the first year, after an allopathic attendant was employed, than during Reichhelm's whole term of a dozen years. And it should be said, the change in medical attendants and modes of practice was owing to the fact that, the control of the institution had passed into the hands of another order of Catholic Sisters, who knew nothing of Homœopathy or preferred a medical attendant of their own religious faith in place of a Lutheran.

When it was discovered that smiles of derision and belittling epithets failed to check the new practice and that those adopting it were not of the poorer and more illiterate classes, nor among those careless of the demands of health, the old physicians became fearful of the competition and adopted new tactics to check its progress. Among other things resorted to was defamation of personal character. On one occasion a slanderous report was circulated by two prominent allopathic physicians, well calculated to utterly ruin the new comer. A respectful but prompt and firm demand for retraction or explanation was made. One of the parties offered a satisfactory explanation and denial, while the other treated the note with contempt. A suit for damages was entered and would have resulted seriously to the traducer but for the interference of his friends who effected a compromise.

So complete was the triumph of our pioneer that the tongue of slander, ever after, touched him lightly and seldom troubled those who came here later as his associates and successors.

For eight years Reichhelm worked on alone, no fellow practitioner coming to his aid till Dr. Charles Bayer located across the river in Allegheny City.

Two years later he had an able and aggressive helper in the person of Dr. D. M. Dake, in this City. Then came Dr. Côté, Dr. Hofmann, Dr. Penniman, and your present orator.

The epidemic of Asiatic cholera, in the year 1849, and its successful treatment by the homœopathic physicians on this field swept away the last great barriers to the acceptance and spread of Homœopathy.

Time would fail me to speak of the subsequent visits of that dread disease, the successes gained in its treatment by our practitioners, the occasional attacks and rejoinders in the public press, the coming of new and able advocates and practitioners, and the rapid increase of friends among the people. The early pioneers have nearly all gone from the field, some to labor in other parts of the county, some to the shades of retirement required by advancing age, and some to the rest, provided in the world now unseen by us, provided for faithful healers of the sick.

Only two or three are left to join with us in celebrating this anniversary.

But, by a wise provision, younger and equally able men are raised up to occupy the field.

It is said to be a fancy peculiar to those grown old in any important line of service, that they imagine when they are gone vacancies will be left that none can fill—that the cause must suffer and the world get wrong. But the faithful historian must record the fact that, in this medical field, the workers of each generation has seemed to have a special fitness for the duties devolving upon them.

Fifty years ago a man of iron mould, cultivated and quick to defend his honor, was demanded.

Reichhelm was finely eductated, of commanding presence, self-reliant, of few words and always cheerful and kind. Those coming after him were better prepared for the polemics of their time, meeting the literary and logical assults of the enemy with the weapons of literature and logic. And those coming later have been more highly endowed with faculties for organizing and building so as to extend professional information through societies, and professional blessings through the dispensary and the hospital.

There are some present, to-day, qualified by a personal acquaintance, to bear witness to the truthfulness of what I have said of Reichhelm and his immediate successors.

EXTENSION OF HOMŒOPATHY.

The spread of the new art of healing, following the lines of what was then the "rapid transit" of the country, extended down the Ohio river.

In 1838 Pulte was in Cincinnati and, the year following, Rosenstein in Louisville.

In 1840 Homœopathy was first known in Indiana; in 1841 in Michigan; in 1842 in Wisconsin; and in 1843 in Illinois, at the "village" of Chicago.

And it affords us great pleasure to have with us, upon this platform to-day, the noble Chicago pioneer and veteran, Dr. David S. Smith, who, besides being the pioneer in our cause, has the distinction of having been longer than any other living man, a practitioner of medicine in the great metropolis of the west.

You will shortly have the privilege of listening to him, as the representative of the city having two flourishing colleges devoted to the therapeutic teachings of Hahnemann, a city so favorably acquainted with Homœopathy that more than half of her taxes are said to be paid by those who depend upon its ministry in times of sickness.

The light of *similia* was seen, the following year, on the Mississippi, at St. Louis, and likewise on the Cumberland, at Nashville. And, so, the work of medical reform, beginning at Pittsburgh, in 1837, spread westward and southward and northward, appearing in Texas and on the Pacific coast just a dozen years after its passage of the Alleghenies.

Its foothold, however, was not so strong, nor its immediate progress so great, at many points, as at Pittsburgh. And it is not strange that it was so; for the pioneers in reformatory movements of any kind, are not all endowed with tact and skill to win success, nor with the necessary steadiness of purpose and perseverance to hold the ground once occupied.

Years elapsed, in some places, before practitioners came who had the requisite endowments.

As already intimated, the greatest help to the spread and entrenchment of Homœopathy in the confidence of the people, in the west (as in most other parts of the civilized world at one time or another) was the prevalence of Asiatic cholera in the years 1849, 1850, 1854, 1866 and 1873.

In a form of disease so well marked, and so destructive of human life, when allowed to take its own way unchecked by therapeutic measures, an opportunity was given for the trial of curative and preventive means, and a comparison of the results.

In this city, in Cincinnati, and in all the cities where cases received homœopathic treatment, the superiority of the new method was most plainly demonstrated.

At no point was this fact disputed except at Cincinnati, where a partisan editor questioned the truthfulness of the reports of cases treated and cured by Drs. Pulte and Ehrmann.

Taking the lists furnished by those gentlemen, an inquiry was instituted from house to house, by a non-medical committee which fully confirmed the homœopathic claims and caused them to be more widely published and to become more convincing than they could otherwise have been.

In the lower Valley of the Mississippi the successes achieved by the practitioners of Homœopathy, in the treatment of the yellow fever, the dreaded scourge of the tropics, have gained the confidence of observing people for the new school and opened every door for its admission. It is generally conceded that cases of Asiatic cholera and yellow fever call for remedies possessed of power rightly to impress the human organism ; and hence our increased number of recoveries must be allowed to mean something.

THE STATE OF MEDICINE FITFY YEARS AGO.

The event we are here to celebrate must take our minds in retrospection to the state of medical art as it appeared fifty years ago in our part of the world. So far as the practice was in pursuance of college teaching—so far as it was not in the hands of our good grandmothers and those accounted as quacks, it was decidedly heroic. The era of calomel, antimony, the blister and the lancet was not gone.

Preventive medicine was little thought of, and the regulation of the air, water, and the food supply for the restoration of health was regarded as quite unbecoming the scientific physician.

The fever patient was kept in a close room, on a feather-bed with few if any changes of linen, and without the refreshing draught of cool water, except where salivation was desired.

Disease, regarded as some mysterious entity, some morbific matter in the blood or stomach or bowels, was to be removed by copious bleedings or by vigorous emetics and cathartics.

With such a crude patholgy and such heroic therapeutics prevalent among our medical men it is little wonder that the reformers, who came denouncing the lancet and the massive and destructive doses of drugs, should be regarded with contempt and met with ridicule. Nor should it be surprising that they were characterized as "fools or knaves."

Gradually the negative good, the fact that more patients with pneumonia, pleurisy, scarlet fever, Asiatic cholera and yellow fever, recovered without bleeding, salivation, blistering or purging, under the mild measures of Homœopathy, led the people to doubt the efficacy and then the safety of the old practice. And the suggestion was not lost on the medical profession. Those who had not arrived at a stage where they are said to "learn nothing and forget nothing," began to take the hint and abandon the heroic measures. And the change among them was hastened by the discovery, that the most enlightened and observing of the people would no longer bear such treatment and were, more and more, resorting to the new practice.

The irreconcilables, those who could "learn nothing and forget nothing," would have been something more than human had they not become alarmed in view of the changes taking place among progressive medical men, as well as among thinking people. They appealed to the coroner, to courts of law and to legislators for the protection of their craft by the repressive force of the civil arm.

In this city, a coroner's inquest and a suit for damages instigated by them, about thirty years ago, against two of our praetitioners, did more to demonstrate the learning and skill on our side of the profession, and the envy and malice on theirs, than years of ordinary controversy and display of clinical proofs could have done. In spite of the learning of a Shaler and the eloquence of a Stanton the result was in our favor.

Though the recollection of such experiences yet lingers with those of us who were on the stage of action here, a third of a century ago, all feelings of resentment and bitterness have passed away. Sustained by public opinion as well as by courts of law, and especially favored by the myriad-tongued press, the great enemy of bigotry and friend of fair dealing and progress, we have held on our way successfully and, to-day, stand in a position to view with composure as well as candor the efforts of all who would place obstacles in our path.

Driven, years ago, to the necessity of organizing societies and schools and establishing journals of our own, we have found in them the way and the power to make ourselves understood and to protect our interests throughout the country; and wisdom admonishes us to adhere to them, till the undoubted right to think on all medical topics and freely to express our thoughts in any society and any medical journal devoted to progress, is conceded on all hands.

It becomes us, however, carefully to guard our own societies, lest the disposition, natural to some orders of mind, to repress new ideas and to place a Chinese wall around doctrines we may cherish to guard them against all change, be allowed to exercise its baneful influence. Any society, devoted to experimental science, which assumes an orthodoxy and directs its energies to the detection and punishment of heterodoxy among its members, has outlived its usefulness and should speedily pass away. Our societies and journals are yet open to the expression of any views, couched in proper terms, from any thinker and any practitioner, be he allopath or homœpath; and when the same freedom and courtesy shall characterize the societies and journals of the old school, then it will do to talk about the dropping of all distinctive titles and all appearances of a separate school. The "trades-union" and "boycotting" methods of our old school friends are not entirely consistent with the claim of being "non-sectarian" and "regular"

THE PRESENT AND FUTURE OF MEDICINE.

Such thoughts bring us to consider the medical field now, as compared with fifty years ago, and to cast our minds forward to fancy the changes yet to come.

In 1837 Reichhelm was the only representative practitioner of the new school west of the Alleghenies, while the year 1887 finds more than five thousand of such practitioners. In every city and town of any importance they are seen to-day, surrounded by clients in all the higher walks of life. A goodly number of coleges have come into existence, and are annually sending out scores of well qualified homœopathic physicians on the western field. State and local societies are numerous and active. Hospitals and dispensaries have been opened to extend the beneficent ministry of *similia* to the suffering poor of the land.

With feelings of pride we must contemplate the progress of homœopathy in this old city, which now, with its sister city across the river and their environs, boasts no less than seventy-five educated medical men devoted to its practice. The Pittsburgh Homœopathic Hospital stands without a superior in this or any other country. It has been my privilege to visit the finest hospitais on both sides of the Atlantic, and I do not hesitate to say that I have nowhere seen one that, in structure, appointment and management, excels that established by the successors of Gustavus Reichhelm and their friends in this city. It will stand, I trust, to commemorate their devotion to truth and humanity long after they, themselves, shall have passed forever from the walks of life.

I must be excused, on this occasion, for some personal references and some expressions of local pride, for it was here I spent years with Reichhelm, first as pupil and then as partner, and finally as successor; and here that I had around me, as students, many bright young men, some of whom have been leading spirits and chief factors in founding and managing the hospital of which I have so proudly spoken. Some of those young men I now see around me—but how changed! The labors of two and three decades, exposure to summer's heat and winter's cold, loss of sleep and harrowing cares have thinned their locks and turned them gray, and laid many a line of earnest thought on brow and cheek.

I am happy, successors, associates and students mine, again to join with you in celebrating the event that has given occupation and field and fortune to you and me, and a most beneficient mode of healing to the great regions of our country lying west of the Allegheny mountains.

THE CENTENNIAL OF THIS EVENT.

When the exercises of this day are closed and we look forward in imagination to an assemblage here to celebrate the hundredth anniversary of the coming of Reichhelm to this city, what is the scene presented? All in this assembly will be gone, save a few of the younger people whose lives may be extended to the "Three score and ten."

The institutions, now comparatively young, will then be looked upon as old; and many will be the changes in the methods and means of the art of healing. I venture to predict the disappearance of hundreds of agents from the materia medica, which are now regarded as useful, sifted out by careful tests and a more critical clinical experience; a better knowledge of the pathogenic and therapeutic influences of the common articles and agencies of life, such as air, water, motion, electricity, food, clothing, occupation and habits; the disappearance of creeds and the distinctions of "orthodoxy" and "heterodoxy" in medicine; and the reign of freedom to think, speak and write in behalf of what each may consider true and best.

The enlightenment brought by the new physiology will make men afraid to cast into the delicate human organism the drugs and doses now regarded as necessary and safe.

So far as internal medication shall be resorted to for the removal of disease, the cure of the sick, aside from gerimicides and palliatives, it will be more or less in obedience to the homœopathic law.

The changes we have seen, during the last fifty years, the abandonment of bleeding, blistering, salivating and endless purging for the cure of the sick, warrants the belief that it will hardly take fifty years to ensure the gentle reign of *similia* throughout our country so far as scientific medicine shall be known.

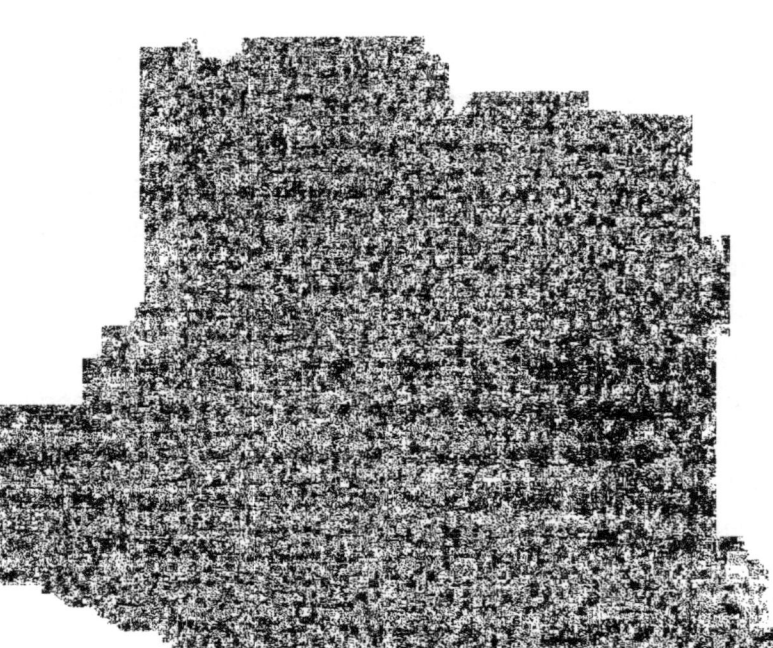

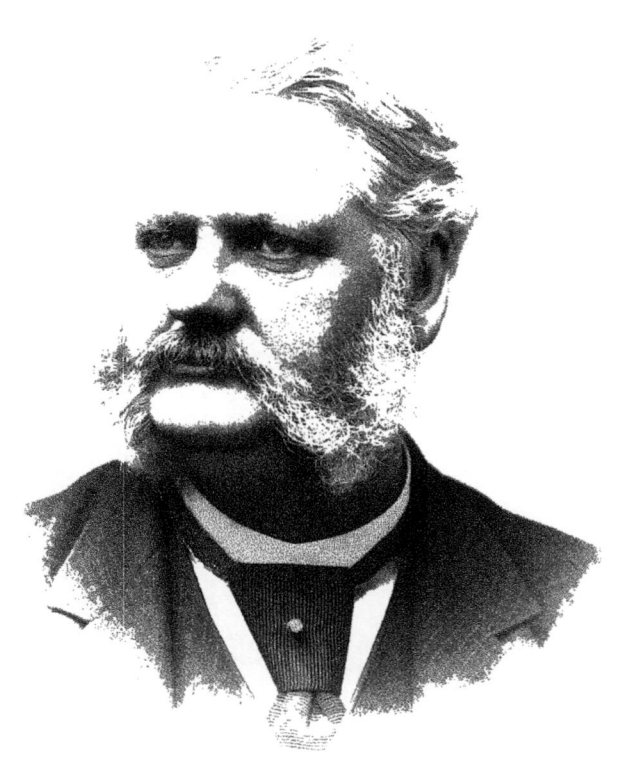

A. R. THOMAS, M. D.

ADDRESS,

By A. R. Thomas, M.D., of Philadelphia, Pa.

Mr. Chairman, Ladies and Gentlemen:

We assemble on this occasion under circumstances of peculiar interest. We celebrate the semi-centennial of the introduction of homœopathy west of the Allegheny Mountains, an event marking an epoch in the history of homœopathy in this country, and one worthy of appropriate commemoration.

As we contemplate the rapid growth and progress made by our school during the past fifty years, noting the increase of the number of practitioners of homœopathy from scarcely 100 in 1837, to probably over 10,000 at the present time; and when we note the rise and progress of our medical colleges, the multiplication of hospitals, dispensaries and of homes and various institutions under our charge, observe the rapid growth of our literature, and remember that while we may not have converted the dominant school, as a body, to our system, we have so modified their methods of practice that blood-letting and salivation, the sheet anchors of the physician fifty years ago, have become quite obsolete, and in their place a mild expectancy generally employed, vastly to the advantage of the poor patients: I say when we remember all this, we may well feel like congratulating ourselves upon what the half century just closed has brought forth.

And when we further reflect upon the world's wonderful progress during the past fifty years; when we consider the marvellous discoveries and inventions; the rapid advance in all the arts and sciences; a progress that has never before been *approximated* in the same period of time, we are led to realize that our lot has been cast in the most interesting and the most eventful period of the world's history.

Fifty years ago the population of the United States was in round numbers but 15,000,000; to-day it reaches over 60,000,000. Within that period our States and Territories have nearly doubled in number. Cities almost without number have sprung into existence and acquired populations of tens and hundreds of thousands. Commerce, manufactures, trade and wealth have increased as by the magic of an Aladdin's lamp. In 1830 there were but 23 miles of railroad in the United States; now we find them forming a vast network over the country, uniting the Atlantic with the Pacific, the North and the South, and giving, in the United States alone over 127,000 miles of track.

Fifty years ago the Mississippi river may be said to have formed the western boundary to the settled portion of our country. The restless tide of emigration has since swept over the great West, and to-day the population west of the Mississippi numbers over 12,000,000, a number four-fifths as great as the population of the whole country in 1837.

But it is not our own country alone that has seen marvellous change in the past fifty years. The old world has passed through revolutions political, social and scientific, scarcely less wonderful. The general employment of steam and electricity has changed the occupations of men, influenced every industry, revolutionized the methods of trade and commerce, and so annihilated time and space as to have made all Europe our next-door neighbors.

While the world has made these rapid advances in material prosperity during the past half century, how has it been with general science and medicine?

Fifty years ago general science was in its merest infancy when compared with its present state. A foundation existed for some sciences, it is true, while others were quite unknown. To quote from a recent author : "In the pride of our hearts we forget how very young science is. We forget how new a power it is in the world, and how feeble and timid was its tender babyhood in the first two decades of the present century. Among the concrete sciences, astronomy, the eldest born, had advanced furthest when our age was still young. But geology had only just begun to emerge from the earliest plane of puerile hypothesis into the period of collection and collocation of facts. Biology, hardly yet known by any better or truer name than natural history, consisted mainly of a jumble of half-classified details. Psychology still wandered disconsolate in the misty domain of the abstract metaphysician. The sciences of man, of language, of society, of religion, had not even begun to exist. The antiquity of our race, the natural genesis of arts and knowledge, and the origin of articulate speech or of religious ideas were scarcely so much as debatable questions. Among sciences of the abstract-concrete class, physics, unilluminated by the clear light of correlation and conservation of energy, embraced a wide and ill-digested mass of separate and wholly unconnected departments. Light had little enough to do with heat, and nothing at all to do in any way with electricity, or sound, or motion, or magnetism. Chemistry still remained very much in the condition of Mrs. Jellaby's cupboard. Everywhere science was tentative and invertebrate, feeling its way on earth with hesitating steps, trying its wings in air with tremulous fear, in preparation for the broader excursions and wider flights of the last three adventurous decades."

Within the period of the present half century, science has extended our knowledge upwards and outwards into the illimitable distances of the universe, as well as downwards in the direction of the infinitesimals of matter and life. New instruments of investigation have been invented, and old ones perfected. The spectroscope, an invention of the recent past, and with the powers of detecting so small a fragment of matter as the $\frac{1}{1000000}$ part of a grain of sodium, has revealed to us the chemical nature, not only of the sun and fixed stars, but to some extent of comets and nebular masses.

The doctrine of the conservation of force, or the convertibility of all forms of energy interchangeably one into the other, is an outgrowth of the present century, a doctrine that has vastly widened and extended our knowledge of the operations of nature and their adaptation to the wants of man.

Not the least of the discoveries of the present age has been that of the potentiality of the infinitesimal. Although, perhaps, not yet generally willing to admit this principle in the action of remedies on the animal organism, yet the scientist recognizes its influence in many operations of nature. He sees it in the upbuilding of reefs, islands and mountains by the almost microscopic coral polyp. The influences that have resulted in the formation of our continents, and given the present conformation to their surfaces, he looks for rather in the action of infinitesimal forces, than in the mighty convulsions of nature to which they were at one time generally attributed. He sees it in the theory, now well established, of the molecular nature and action of matter, while with microscope and spectroscope, his studies are directed as much to the infinitesimals of nature, as to her grosser developments. The etiologist and pathologist of the present day find, associated with many diseases, certain minute organisms, vegetable or animal, the microbes or bacilli of the present time, and which, whether bearing the relation to disease of cause or effect, become interesting illustrations of the infinitesimal in the pathological processes of the body. The influence of all this is directly calculated to prepare the way for the more ready and general acceptance of an essential doctrine of homœopathy —the action of remedies in infinitesimal doses.

Then the advance made in electrical science during the past half century has been something truly wonderful. Fifty years ago electricity was seldom referred to except as an interesting scientific curiosity. Of its relation to galvanism and magnetism, little or nothing was known, while of its wonderful physical and therapeutic powers we were wholly ignorant. The only attempt at the useful control of the power was in the employment of the lightning rod. Since, in addition to the telegraph with its vast influence upon the world, electrical science has given us the wonderful telephone and microphone. Electric lights are seen everywhere, and electricity has become a motor power threatening to supplant all others.

In the beginning of the present half century (1839) the daguerrotype appeared. Later came the photograph, followed by numerous improvements, and by various processes for the reproduction of pictures, until to-day, this branch of art has reached a degree of perfection never dreamed of fifty years ago.

Of the many scientific developments of the past fifty years, that which has perhaps attracted the widest attention, and given rise to the most heated controversies, that has more than any other tended to revolutionize all our views of the great questions of nature and man, is the doctrine of evolution. Although foreshadowed by some of the writers of the latter part of the past, and the beginning of the present century, it has been within the past thirty years that the doctrine has been clearly formulated and presented to the world.

Embodying, as it does, vastly more than the theory of the origin of species and the descent of man as given by Darwin, evolution, as taught by the latter, with Huxley, Spencer, Lubbock and others, deals with universal nature. Looking far backward, it sees the whole physical universe as starting in the remote past from a diffuse and probably nebulous condition, in which all matter, reduced to a state of extreme tenuity, occupied an incomprehensibly wide area of space.

Of our own solar system, evolution teaches us to regard the sun with its attendant planets and their several satellites, all in their several orbits, as owing their shape, size, relations and movements, not to external design and deliberate creation, but to the slow and regular working out of physical laws, in accordance with which, each has assumed its existing weight and bulk and path and position.

In the organic world, without attempting to account for the origin or source of life, evolution seeks to trace the gradual development of higher from lower forms, through the vegetable to the animal, and from lower animal forms, slowly up to man; the influence of environment, heredity, the struggle for existence, with the survival of the fittest, being the great factors operating to gradually bring about the present condition of the organic world. Whatever missing links there may be in the chain of evidences for the support of this doctrine, however repugnant it may be to our sense of the dignity of man, however the theory may conflict with our earlier teachings upon this subject, evolution, nevertheless, has been received with such a degree of favor by the scientific world, that there can be no question as to the permanency of its endurance.

While the world has been making such vast strides in general progress; while discovery, invention, the arts and sciences, and all knowledge have been making such wonderful advance, how has it been with medicine? What was the condition of general medicine in 1837 when Gustavus Reichhelm entered this city as a pioneer of the new system of therapeutics? The late Professor

Gross,* in his recently published autobiography, says: "When I entered the profession fifty years ago, it was covered with a mantle of darkness. Theories, conjectures and uncertainties were the characteristics of the day. Hardly anything was definitely settled. Physiology and pathology were conjectural branches of the healing art. Chemistry was in a rudimentary transitional state. Hygiene and state medicine had no existence. Toxicology and medical jurisprudence were occult arts. Surgery and medicine were the merest arts, without any scientific associations or connections. Midwifery and gynecology were in a most crude condition. Disease was by many regarded, not as an aberration of function, or perversion of health, but a sort of undefined entity engrafted upon the system, from which it was necessary to expel it, often with violent remedies more injurious to the patient than the malady itself. Therapeutics had been more labored than advanced. Very little was certainly known respecting the action of remedies upon the system. The text books were of an inferior order, and medical literature had made little progress."

The above is no doubt a fair statement of the condition of general medicine fifty years ago. But now how changed! Indeed the past half century has seen more advance in the progress of general medical science than in any previous equal period in the world's history. The discovery of the power and use of the several anæsthetics, the greatest boon to suffering humanity which the age has produced, has not only saved a vast amount of suffering, but has rendered possible the performance of operations never before attempted, and has thus led to an advance in operative surgery which could never have been otherwise attained.

---

*Samuel D. Gross, M.D., Professor of Surgery in the Jefferson Medical College, Philadelphia, Pa.

The employment of antisepsis in both medicine and surgery, so much in vogue within a few years, has already given wonderful results. In the great lying-in hospitals of Vienna, Dresden and other large cities of Europe, through the strict antiseptic precautions employed, the mortality has been reduced from 18 to 20 per cent. to almost nothing. Fifty years ago the average of human life in Great Britain was thirty years, while according to recent statistics it is at the present time forty-nine years. Within the same period of time the population of Great Britain has increased 8,000,000, and of this number 2,000,000 are claimed as the direct result of better sanitary conditions, and of victory over preventable diseases. With his antiseptic methods, the surgeon performs his most extensive operations—amputates limbs and breasts, removes tumors, opens the abdominal cavity, and applies his dressings with the greatest assurance of finding, upon their removal at the end of six to ten days, a perfect healing with perhaps not a drop of pus. When we remember with what hesitation and dread the abdominal cavity was opened but a few years ago, wounding of the peritoneum being looked upon as attended in every case with the utmost danger; and that the healing of the parts after nearly every operation was attended by extensive suppuration and a slow process of granulation, I say when we remember this and compare it with the results attained to-day, we may begin to realize the vast progress of the but recent past, and to appreciate something of the possibilities of the future.

Medical education has also made great advancement during the past half century. Less than fifty years ago, five to seven professors, with a single demonstrator, constituted the whole teaching body in the best schools in the country. Anatomy and Physiology, or Surgery and Obstetrics, or perhaps Anatomy and Surgery, were frequently taught from the same chair. Pathology,

Morbid Anatomy, Histology and Sanitary Science had no place in the medical curriculum. The student got no practical work whatever, except in the dissecting room, saw but little clinical medicine or surgery, and after two short courses of three or four months of annually repeated lectures, was deemed competent to assume the great responsibilities of the healing art. How different is it to-day! We find in the best schools the curriculum greatly widened, the course prolonged to six or more months, the teaching body increased to twenty, twenty-five and even thirty or more; and instead of the old and illogical method, in which the student on his first day in college, listened not only to lectures on the rudimentary branches, as anatomy, physiology and chemistry, but at the same time upon obstetrics, practice and surgery, subjects that he was totally unprepared to comprehend, we now have the graded course of three years, in which the student first takes up the fundamental branches, followed by the practical and special.

In view of the great progress of medicine during the more recent past, what may we expect of the future? That the development of our art is to continue, and that improvements no less important than those of the past are certain to be developed, none can doubt. Dark points in physiology are to be cleared up. Etiology and pathology are to be better understood. New operations and new methods in surgery are to give better results. But it is without doubt, in the direction of *preventive medicine* and *therapeutics*, that we are to look for the great developments of the future. Our increasing knowledge of zymotic diseases, with a better acquaintance with the origin, methods of propagation, and means of distribution of the microscopic germs inducing them, must ultimately lead to the discovery of the means for the control, if not for the complete prevention of these several diseases.

The great aim and ultimate object of the medical sciences being that of relieving human suffering and prolonging life, therapeutics, which has directly to do with the cure of disease and for which all other branches of the science but form a foundation, becomes the very cap-stone of the temple of medicine. Anatomy has made us thoroughly familiar with the structure of the human body; physiology has taught us the use of the various parts and organs; etiology has given us a vast amount of information as to the cause and source of the majority of our diseases, while pathology and morbid anatomy have acquainted us with the progress and structural changes resulting from morbid processes. But without a system of therapeutics, without power to successfully combat and control disease, all this knowledge becomes of little practical value. Hence, the importance of this subject in the medical curriculum. While therapeutics may not have kept pace with other branches of medicine in the past, it has nevertheless made great advance within the past century. The doctrine of Hahnemann has not only resulted in the formation of a new school of medicine, but its influence has admittedly vastly modified the practice of the old. Seeing our success with small doses, they have been led to halt in their career of heroic medication, and in its place we find either a mild expectancy, or so little faith in any medication, that we are told by Dr. Holmes that, "with the exception of opium, quinine and perhaps a few other remedies, it would be better for the sick if all the medicine in the world were thrown into the sea, and so much the worse for the fishes." The complicated polypharmacy of the past has been wonderfully modified. Of the multitude of samples with which the office table of the physician of the present day will be found covered, it is a notable fact, that in nearly every case, the article is a *simple* one; rarely will a compound be seen.

In the law of similars as developed by Hahnemann we claim to possess a key to the solution of the great question of therapeutics, a guide for the treatment of all curable diseases, by following which, we may cure our cases more safely, more rapidly and more scientifically.

But we are led to inquire, are there no other means or methods or aids, that may be employed in the treatment of disease? Does homœopathy constitute the whole of therapeutical science? Is the physician best prepared to cope with disease in its varied forms, whose knowledge and use of drugs is always and only confined to their homœopathic use? Has the physician discharged his full duty to his patient in all cases, when he has made the most careful selection and administration of the closest similimum of the symptoms of the case? May the medical school, in view of its responsibility in the education of physicians, confine its therapeutical teachings to the homœopathic medication alone? These are important questions, and the future of homœopathy to no small degree will depend upon their solution. Therapeutics, being the science of healing, embraces *everything* that may in any way aid in the restoration of health to the sick or injured. Thus, mechanical measures constitute the principal therapeutical means employed by the surgeon. Without his knife and numerous instruments and apparatus, he would be almost powerless in the treatment of surgical cases. *Antidotal* therapeutics will be required in the treatment of cases of poisoning. *Hydro* and *electro*-therapeutics may be made great aids in the treatment of many diseases, while the employment of *palliative* therapeutics often becomes an important duty. But we are sometimes told that the true and loyal homœopathic physician will, and should, have nothing to do with palliative medication. The inconsistency of such a position is easily established. What would we think of the surgeon who, under such a claim, should refuse to employ anæsthetics in his operations, subjecting his patients to the needless agony of the cruel knife? We would designate him a monstrous fanatic. If the employment of anæsthetics is justifiable on the part of the surgeon, no less so is the use of anodynes or other palliatives on the part of the physician, in the management of many cases of incurable or other diseases attended with great pain and suffering.

It is admitted that the employment of such measures may be attended in some cases, with a degree of risk, and always with some danger of abuse. So much *more* important does it become therefore, that the student should be thoroughly and carefully instructed in everything relating to this subject. Fully informed as to the action of palliative medicines, carefully instructed as to their indications or contra-indications, cautioned as to their danger and watchful of their effects, he is in a far better position for discharging the duties of the honest physician, than he who repudiates all such measures, or ignorantly resorts to their use.

But you may tell me that students so instructed will be in danger of becoming eclectics, or of going over to the old school, and abandoning homœopathy entirely. I reply that if the success of homœopathy is depending upon keeping her students ignorant upon all of these important subjects, if to give them a broad and liberal education is at the risk of their deserting our ranks, then is our hold upon them weak indeed, and the days of homœopathy are nearly numbered. On the contrary, if our system of practice is ever to acquire that power and influence in the medical world that has so long been predicted for it, it must and *can* be accomplished only by our medical schools imparting to their students the most thorough and complete instruction in *every* branch of medical science. Upon the medical schools of the present and future there rests, therefore, a heavy responsibility. They must keep step with the rapid march of every department of science. The curriculum of study must be frequently widened. The requirements for matriculation must be made more exacting and the final examinations more rigid. The didactic lectures must be supplemented by practical laboratory work in all the practical branches. They must be supplied with apparatus, both physical, chemical and surgical, and with a museum of anatomy, both normal and pathological, ample for the illustration and demonstration of every subject. A fully equipped hospital must be under their management and control, that the student may enjoy abundant opportunity for clinical instruction in every branch or specialty of medicine and surgery. In short, the medical colleges must be prepared to supply the constantly increasing demand for *thoroughly* and *liberally* educated *physicians*, in the widest acceptance of those terms.

But the responsibility in this matter does not rest alone with the faculties of the medical colleges. The profession at large, and the general public, have duties in this direction as well. The profession should be ready to second every movement of the colleges for advancement, and should stand ready to assist in their accomplishment. They should encourage only the best talent to engage in the study. They should see to it that their students shall not, with the view of saving a few dollars, or of securing their diploma in a shorter period, wander off to the shorter term and poorly equipped institutions. If the profession of the country, really and earnestly desire a higher grade of general and scientific education for their students, they have only to encourage and support those already struggling for the attainment of that end, and they will soon accomplish their purpose.

It is the duty of the public at large, for the benefit of which medical schools are directly laboring, to encourage and support by a liberal contribution of their abundance for the endowment of medical colleges, and for the erection and support of hospitals, the two at the present day being inseparably connected. To what nobler purpose can the surplus means of the wealthy be appropriated? Not only is the present generation benefited, but the beneficent results may be made to extend through all coming time.

I have referred to the marvelous discoveries and inventions, and to the wonderful advance in general and medical sciences made during the past half century. What will the next fifty years bring forth? The most active imagination would probably fall far short of the truth in an attempt to picture the reality. Without further venturing into the field of prophecy, we will leave the facts to be recorded by the historian of the *centennial* of the event we this day celebrate.

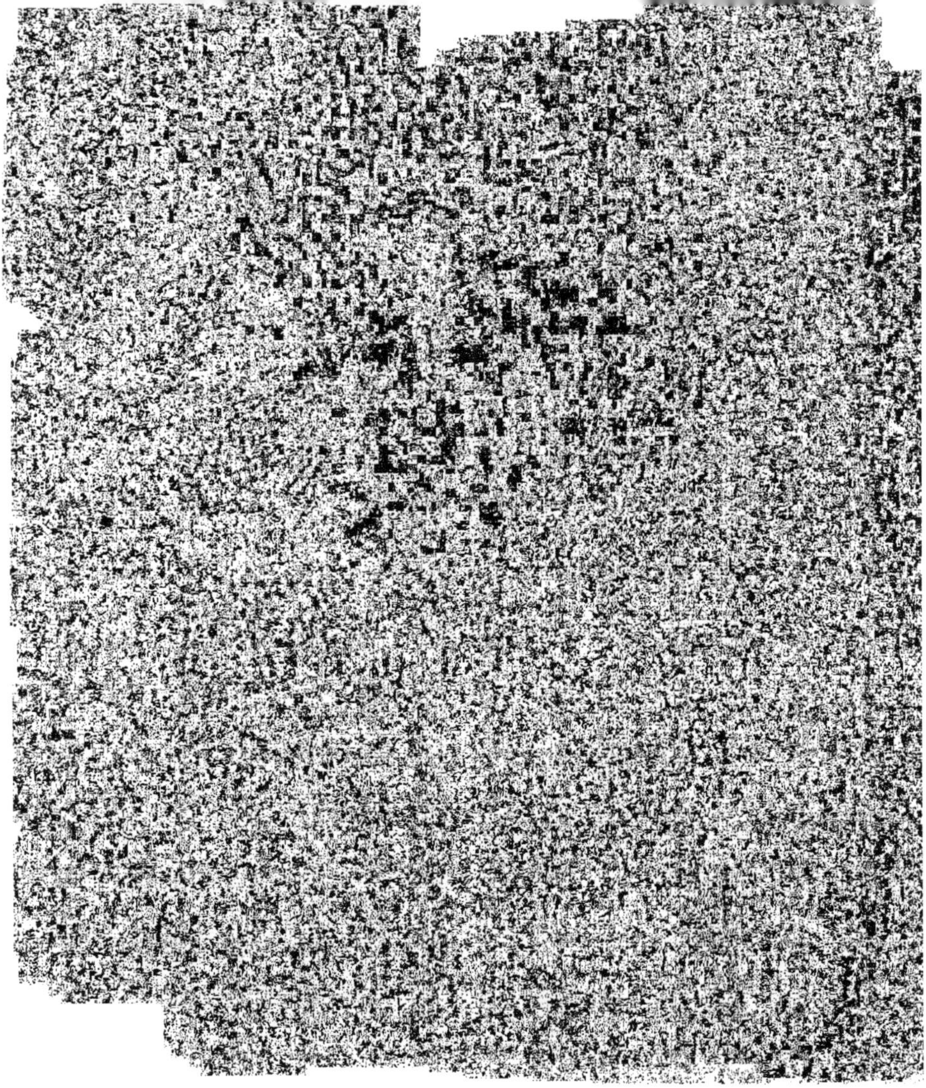

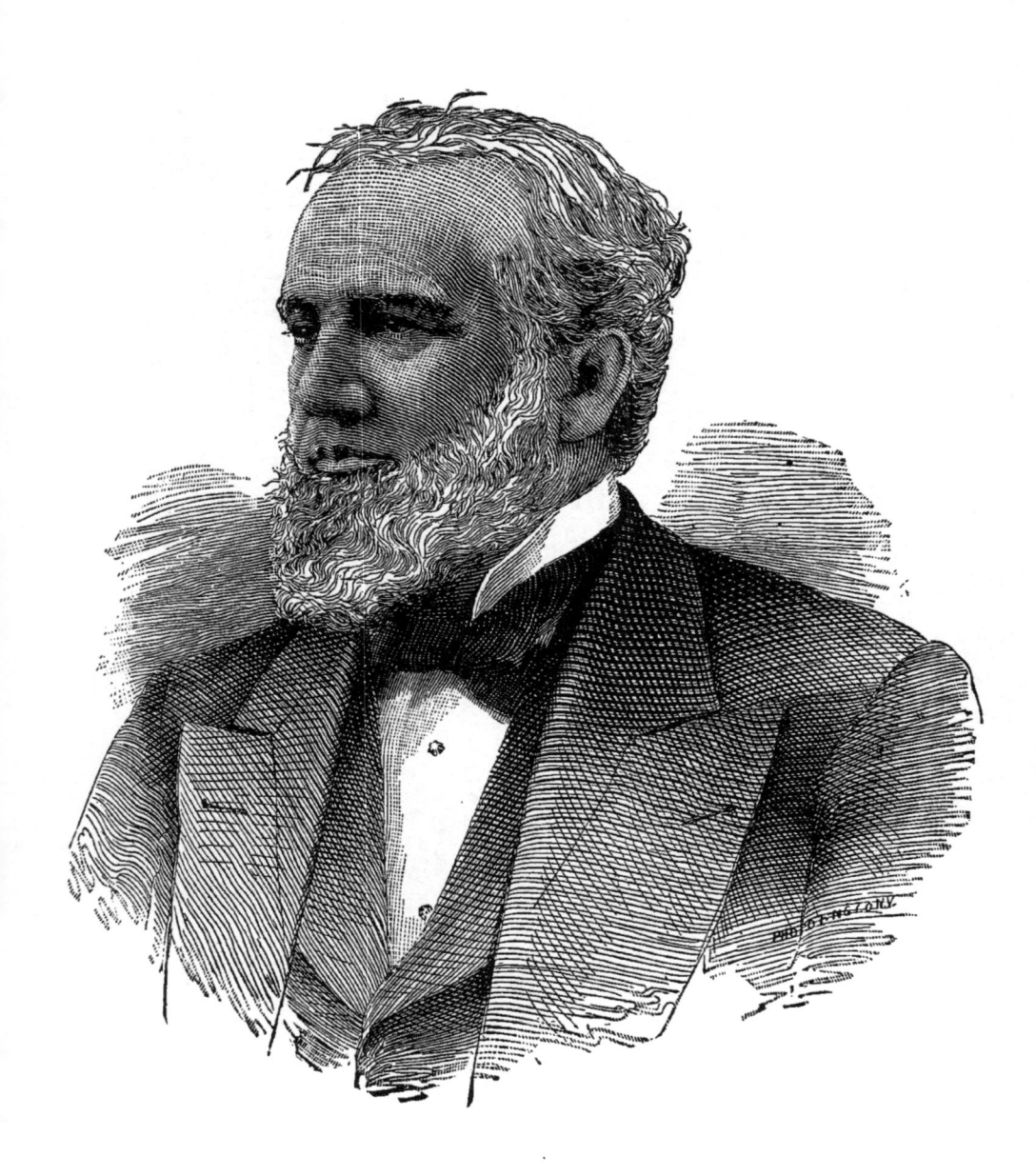

D. S. SMITH, M. D.

ADDRESS,

By D. S. Smith, M.D., of Chicago, Ill.

Mr. Chairman, Ladies and Gentlemen :

Although I appear before you without notes, manuscript or preparation, I most gladly join with you in this semi-centennial celebration of the advent of Homœopathy west of the picturesque Allegheny Mountains, whose summits I crossed fifty years ago a full fledged Allopath.

Early in the spring of 1836 I left my home in Camden, N. J., with my diploma from the Jefferson Medical College of Philadelphia. My objective point being Chicago, I stopped on my way in this city, which, even at that remote time, gave evidence of the future greatness, which is now being so fully realized as the great manufacturing city of iron and glass, and at this time the development of natural gas, is changing its complexion, making its atmosphere clean and the city itself more desirable for residence. After some delay and many regrets at leaving this enterprising city, I continued my way to Chicago, reaching there in May, where I at once opened an office for the practice of my profession. There I found few physicians, in fact, few were needed, as Chicago then counted its population at about three thousand. Their practice in the treatment of disease was heroic to the extreme, as illustrated by their administration of calomel from twenty to eighty grains at one dose, and their free use of drastic pills and emeto-cathartics, to meet the demands of a restless, active people, who would not wait for the *vis medica-*

trix naturæ, but who wanted a prompt, effective medicine to "kill or cure," and unfortunately it was not always a cure. Esthetics were not as much considered in the arrangement of our offices in those early days, neither were our libraries as extensive as we find them in this decade.

Being in Philadelphia in the winter of 1837-38, I had occasion during the serious illness of my child to call in my preceptor, a distinguished physician of those days. He gave as his opinion that the disease was constitutional and recovery very doubtful. The child failing to improve, I consulted another professor famed for his successful treatment of children, and he expressed an opinion similar to that of my preceptor. At the solicitations of friends who were firm believers in the Homœopathic school of medicine, I was induced to get such medicines and books as I could then procure, Hahnemann's Organon and Jahr's Manual as translated by Dr. Hering. Under the Homœopathic medication which I then gave, the child soon recovered.

I returned to Illinois in the spring of 1838 and commenced prescribing Homœopathic remedies, and continued to do so, but without especial publicity. In the spring of 1843 I went to New York, where I gave attention to this school of practice, and procured all the works on the subject I could there find printed in English; also, a more extensive supply of medicines. Among the books that I then obtained were the first edition of "Hull's Jahr," "Jahr's Manual of Homœopathic Practice," and these works were very serviceable to me, and to this day I would by no means be satisfied if my library did not contain Jahr's Manual.

Thus armed I commenced work in earnest. The success which then followed aroused much criticism and opposition among my Allopathic friends, who thus aided me in bringing before the public this new science of therapeutics, and having a great truth to demonstrate, the victory was ours as is evidenced to-day by the growth of Homœopathic practice in Chicago and throughout the great Northwest. It even extended to the Pacific coast, and even the Pacific did not stay its progress. At that time to my certain knowledge, I was the only practicing Homœopathist west of the great lakes. We then had some very distinguished laymen in our city—the late Hon. Wm. B. Ogden, the late Hon. Thomas Hoyne and the Hon. P. Y. Scammon. These gentlemen were active friends of our cause, and the latter is to-day one of the Trustees of the Hahnemann Medical College and Hospital, of Chicago. In those early days of Homœopathy the editors of the daily papers rendered us efficient service in permitting us the use of their columns, and I take pleasure in acknowledging the kindly aid of the public press, which is always ready to advance any good or noble cause.

The oration of Wm. Cullen Bryant, delivered in 1841 before the New York State Homœopathic Society, was published in one of our papers, and subsequently in pamphlet form, and circulated extensively in the city and throughout that region of country. The circulation of this pamphlet I consider rendered our cause good service. Then, as now, there were some high minded honorable gentlemen among the Allopathists, who, while differing from us, were willing to accord to others what they claimed for themselves, namely, a right to think and act according to their convictions.

The "Northwestern Journal of Homœopathy" appeared about this time, followed later by a bi-monthly for the general reader, with a two-fold mission. One was to popularize the new system, and the other to bring before the community and the profession a couple of young physicians who had recently arrived in our city. One of these soon crossed the dark river, and the other has gained a reputation which has extended over two continents. He would have been here to-day had not his duties as Dean of the Hahnemann College detained him there at the opening exercises for the winter. This monthly having accomplished its mission ceased in 1856. Next "The Investigator" was published. Following that came "The United States Medical and Surgical Journal," edited by several medical gentlemen of our city. It was an able exponent of the principles and practice of Homœopathy. Since then other similar journals have from time to time made their appearance doing good service in the cause of Homœopathy.

The American Institute of Homœopathy was organized in 1844, and local societies have been extending throughout the several States. Our own city is keeping step in the march of progress. The Northwest, making Chicago its central point, leads with two colleges. There is one in Missouri, one in Iowa, one in Minnesota, one in California, and there may even be others which my memory fails to note. These several colleges, I have reason to believe, are doing a good work, all contributing to meet the great demand made by the cities and villages throughout the great Northwest for good in educating Homœopathic physicians.

In conclusion we have the demonstration of the superiority of the grand truths and principles of Homœopathy in the fact that within the professional life of one man, from less than a half dozen physicians west of the Alleghenies, we now have them numbering many thousands, their locations extending even to the "Golden Gates" and the islands of the great Pacific Ocean.

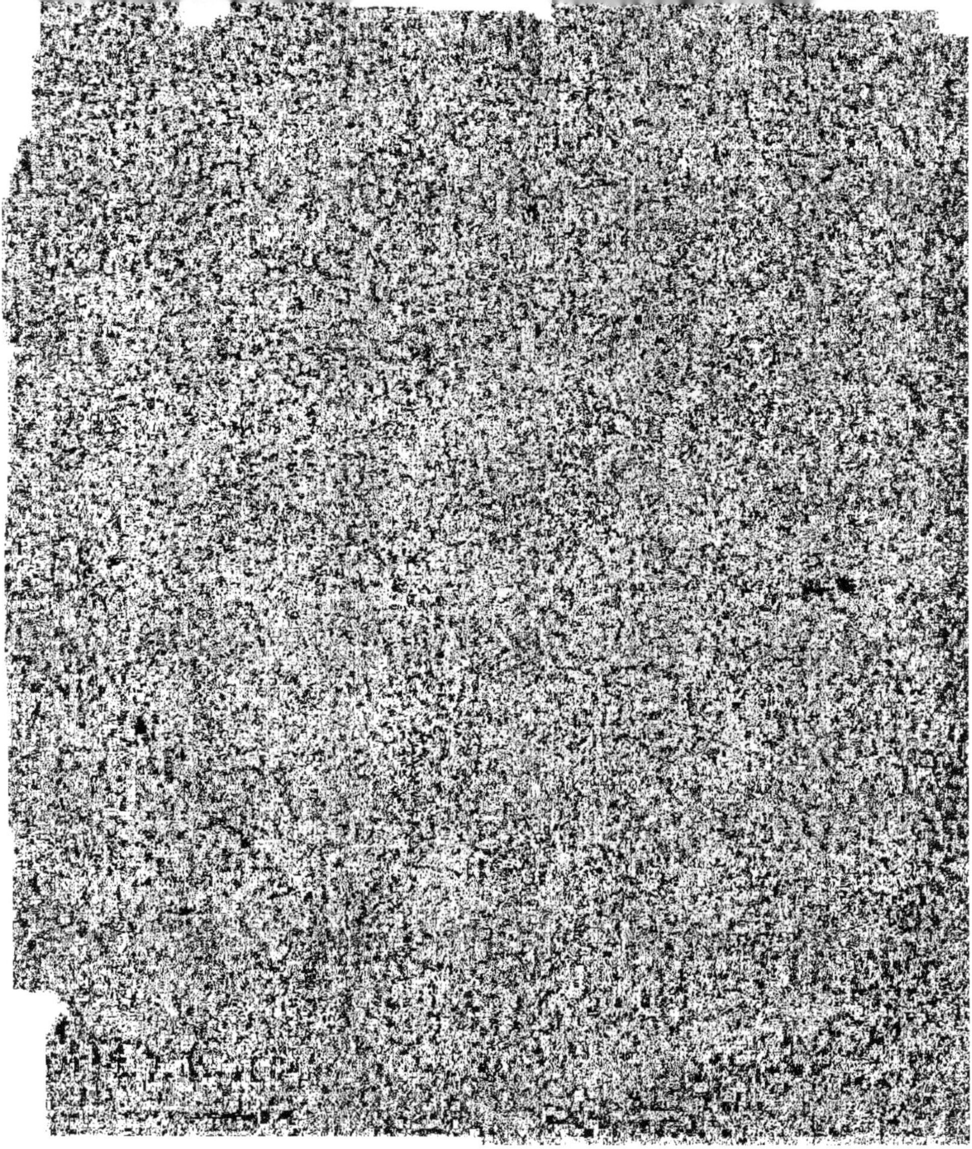

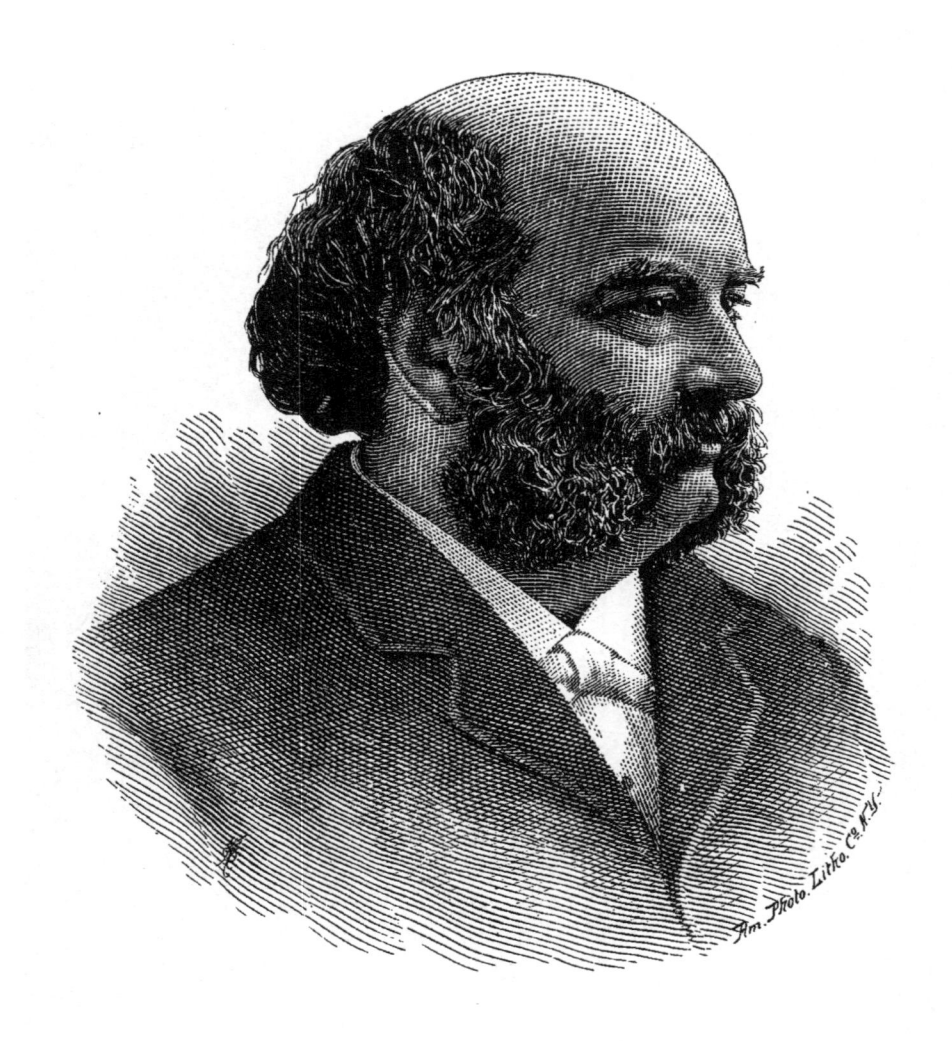

J. W. Dowling, M. D.

ADDRESS,

By J. W. Dowling, M.D., of New York City, N. Y.

Mr. Chairman, Ladies and Gentlemen:

In the invitation extended to me to be present and participate in the exercises—the festivities of this day—I am requested by your committee to say a few words on medicine in this country as compared with that of fifty years ago. Before entering upon my subject, which I shall consider briefly, I must congratulate you, members of the Homœopathic Medical Society of Allegheny County, and the friends of our school in this section, on the position which Homœopathy occupies right here—on the completion of your magnificent hospital, and on the fact that your society has solved the vexed question of qualification for the practice of medicine, by resolving to admit no young men or women as students in your offices till they have passed a satisfactory examination by a committee from your body, as to their preliminary education and fitness for the *study* of the now many and intricate branches—sciences—connected with the healing art.

If the various medical societies of the country would adopt, and carry out, as you have done, a similar course, there would be no occasion for preliminary examinations at our medical colleges, and legislation on the subject of medicine by our various State Assemblies would be unnecessary.

Not long since, in a conversation which I had with a distinguished physician of our school, he remarked: "Look at Pittsburgh; see the strides they are making there." I replied: "Do you refer to their iron furnaces?" He answered, "No." "To the coal production in that section?" "No." "To the introduction and utilization of their natural gas?" He answered, "No; I refer to the strides which Homœopathy has made,—to the honest labors of the Homœopathic physicians of Pittsburgh. This semi-centennial celebration is an evidence of all this, and my firm belief is that at your centennial anniversary Homœopathy will be the universal method of practice, not only in your own city, but throughout the civilized world. Some of us older ones will long before that time have been laid to rest, but many within the sound of my voice will live to see our law of cure acknowledged as the only law by which curable diseases may be cured, and incurable diseases made comparatively easy for sufferers to bear.

I took it for granted, when I learned that the Grand Opera House had been selected as your meeting place to-day, that the audience would be made up partially, perhaps largely, of laymen and women. I propose addressing my remarks to them. I can say nothing on the subject of ancient and modern medicine which is not already known to the members of the medical profession present to-day, but the laity know little about medicine. They often think they do, but they do not. Some may have a little knowledge of the art, but a little knowledge of medicine is worse than no knowledge at all, and unless you propose to devote your lives to the unceasing study of the healing art, do not try to *unravel its mysteries.* "*For that are we doctors.*" But it will do you no harm for me to tell you briefly what medicine once was, and then compare with what it now is.

The late Wendel Philips, in his lecture on "The Lost Arts,"

contended that in nearly every science the ancients were the equals of the present generation, and from his conclusive arguments you would be led to believe that all recent discoveries are, in reality, merely revivals of sciences and arts long since temporarily lost to the world. On the subject of medicine he was silent. Perhaps in those days there was such an advanced state of civilization that no such science was required,—that doctors, men and women, were not needed. For it is contended at the present day by many intelligent men, that health depends upon conditions which, if observed, will render medicine unnecessary. In the language of one distinguished writer, health depends upon diet, exercise, sleep, the state of the mind, and the state of the atmosphere, and upon nothing else. The ancients may have been able to regulate all of these to their own satisfaction. Where I live we can not do it, and even here, almost in the shadow of those glorious old mountains, you sometimes have, if the papers tell the truth, financial and other disturbances which take away your appetites, perhaps render you unable to gratify them, render you unable to take exercise, disturb your minds, keep you from sleeping nights, and make the atmosphere of your town more smoky than it was when I hurriedly passed through a few years ago, prior to the substitution of your natural gas for bituminous coal. With the revival of civilization, and the lost arts, people did want doctoring; perhaps they required it. *Many*, even in these days, want it who *do not* require it, and they get it, too. If they did not, the doctors would starve.

The oldest work on medicine which I have had the pleasure of perusing, was published in the year 1598, nearly three hundred years ago. I have been much amused and interested in perusing its pages. It is evidently one of the earliest books on this subject published in the English language, for in its introduction it reads: "Until within a recent period the sick were placed in the streets and highways that all passing and repassing might behold them, and seeing that poor, afflicted soul in such a miserable and lamentable state, themselves having had the same disease at divers and sundry times, might the better and easier participate unto the patient the means whereby *they* recovered and attained unto their pristinate and accustomed health; and because in their times, also in the self-same way, all sick and diseased persons might, through the mercy and will of God, be of their maladies cured. And that all might be cured of their maladies, these rules for the cure of the sick have been, through many excilent and God-inspired men, compacted and compiled together in this perfection and excellency." And then as a prelude to the work, the author says, very sensibly, too: " A true physician must first of all know, before he may employ himself to the practice of physic, to wit: that he not only must properly and very well know the complexions of the sick, his strength, age, his affairs and manner of living, but also the sickness itself, with all the circumstances thereof." And without giving the slightest information as to how this knowledge is to be acquired, he commences his prescriptions for certain troubles, the first of which, in the index, is, "A capital corroboration, which is very excilent." The next, which must have been very valuable, is "A good confection for an imbecile head," then "A most excilent water for the head, called the Emperor Charles, his water, which will certainly fortify and corroborate the memory." We have needed some of that water in New York lately. This decoction consists of some twenty or thirty different ingredients which must be mixed and prepared at certain seasons of the year, and then to accomplish the wonderful result must be snuffed through the nostrils.

" We have excilent remedies for the sudden striking of God's hand," by which I suppose the author means modern apoplexy.

"One of the best remedies recommended for this is asses blood, especially blood of a miller's ass, which must be taken out of the ear of the animal; dose, three drops three times daily, and with God's aid he will recover the use of his members." And then we have an excellent water for the naughty scabies, and an unguent for the same, consisting of pulverized brimstone and fresh butter, which is used at the present day for the same condition.

We have a precious remedy for the restoration of the sight, composed of pulverized crickets, with which the eye is to be annointed. This remedy is said to have restored the sight of the Archduke Frederick after a total blindness of seven years duration. Next is an excellent, most true and tried remedy for sterility. Also a purgative powder, consisting of young nettles and the buds of elder. We have also the balm of the poor little unborn infants.

This author was certainly more considerate in his prescriptions to the poor than physicians of the present day. For he has remedies for the poor and others for the rich, suffering from the same disease.

In one instance, the refuse or the barn-yard in a decoction of cinnamon water is prescribed for a *poor* woman suffering from certain conditions. Following this is another for rich folks, the component parts of which are white amber, coral, white and blue sapphires, pickerels eyes and teeth, harts bones, and filings of gold, which must be pulverized together and administered in drachm doses. This work is made up of just such prescriptions, many of them inert in their character, possessing the quality which has been attributed to our Homœopathic remedies, of being, to say the least, harmless. Patients recovered then, as they do now, under the mind cure and other innocent measures, and the doctor received the credit. If they died, everything had been done within the power of man,—it was by the will of God.

We will skip over the period of time intervening between this and the beginning of the present century, and give you in a few words examples of the treatment of the sick a few decades ago by the so-called regular physicians, before the introduction of Homœopathy, and compare this treatment with that of the so-called regular school of the present day, and then simply ask the question, "Has Homœopathy had anything to do with this wonderful change?" I never hear this word *regular* applied to the old school of medicine without a mental or an audible protest. It does not properly apply. Nothing could be more irregular than the regular practice of fifty years ago,—yes, of to-day. They have no regular guide, no law, it is medicine of experiment, then of experience. Even at the recent International Congress, held at Washington, the chairman of the section in therapeutics advanced a new theory as to the action of remedial agents. When the practitioners of the old school learn that when their remedies cure disease—radically cure it, they do so by the law of similars—the so-called Homœopathic law—and endeavor to practice in accordance with that law, they will become *regular* practitioners of medicine. Until then their practice is uncertain and largely experimental, and they are irregular practitioners.

We have learned something of ancient medicine, at least so far back as we are able to trace it. Let us see what regular medicine was fifty years ago. A physician is called to a case of pneumonia or pleurisy. He refers to his authorities; he finds the following advice laid down: "Begin with a large and free bleeding, not deterred by the obscure pulse sometimes found in peri-pneumonia, carrying this evacuation to faintness; repeating these bleedings as the strength of the patient will bear.

Application of a blister to the chest. Antimony combined with mercury, must be administered. Opium to allay the cough and to procure sleep. Squills in nauseating, even emetic doses, to relieve the patient from the viscid matter collected in the air passages."

Carditis and pericarditis, treatment the same as that of pneumonia: "Free bleeding, a blister over the heart, purging to a greater extent than in pneumonia, opium to procure sleep."

Meningitis: "Begin on the first attack of the disease by bleeding the patient as largely as his strength will permit. In some instances it may be productive of more relief if the temporal artery or jugular vein be opened. Cupping and leeches in the progress of the complaint; active cathartics given directly after taking blood; calomel with jalap, antimonial and mercurial preparations; blisters to the back of the neck, behind the ears, and to the temples; mustard poultice to the feet."

Croup: "Blood from the arm or jugular vein; several leeches along the fore part of the neck; a nauseating emetic; ipecacuaha with tartarized antimony, cathartics, diaphoretics, digitalis to control the heart's action; large blisters near the affected part; mercury to speedy salivation; opium," etc.

This is what was called the antiphlogistic treatment, those medicines, plans of diet, etc., which tend to oppose inflammation, or which, in other words, weaken the system by diminishing the activity of the vital power. And so I could go on and enumerate every inflammatory disease, and would find by consulting the authors of fifty,—yes, thirty years ago, this same debilitating system of torture was recommended.

Is it any wonder, with this universal treatment, together with the starving process called the antiphlogistic diet, that these inflammatory diseases were dreaded; that patients feared placing themselves in the hands of the physician, and that they should expect a three weeks' or a month's sickness, dating from the first visit made by their medical attendant?

Is it to be wondered at that sensible men should have looked with distrust, with suspicion, upon the so-called science of medicine, and that they should have advised the throwing of physic to the dogs? Was this an improvement on the system of three hundred years ago, when the mind of the patient was the principal medium through which the physician worked his cure, sensible enough to leave the disease to the tender care of nature? Is it surprising that physicians should have been accused of destroying valuable lives, which, had it not been for their treatment, would have recovered from their ailments? Is it a wonder that Addison should have laid it down as a maxim, "That when a nation abounds in physicians it grows thin of people."

Napoleon I. was not a believer in the practice of physic then in vogue, and once said to his chief physician: "Believe me, we had better leave off all these remedies; life is a fortress that you and I know nothing about. Why throw obstacles in the way of its defense? Its own means are superior to all the apparatus of your laboratory. Medicine is a collection of uncertain prescriptions, the results of which, taken collectively, are more fatal than useful to mankind." The celebrated Zimmerman went from Hanover to attend Frederick the Great in his last illness. One day the King said to him, "You have, I presume, sir, helped many a man into another world." The doctor replied, "Not so many as your majesty, nor with such honor to myself."

Medical practice was defined in those days to be, for the most part, guessing at nature's intentions and wishes, and then endeavoring to substitute man's. Nature, says a French philosophical writer, is "fighting with disease—a blind man armed with a club, that is the physician, steps in to settle the difficulty.

He first, to his credit, tries to make peace. When he cannot accomplish this, he lifts his club and strikes at random. If he strikes the disease, he kills the disease; if he strikes nature, he kills the patient."

A celebrated physician, after conducting a prominent practice for thirty years, retired from the profession, giving as his reason that he was weary of guessing.

The death of Pope Adrian occasioned such joy in Rome that the night after his decease they adorned the door of his chief physician's house with garlands, adding this inscription: "To the deliverer of his country."

No man seems to have had a better knowledge of the workings of this so-called regular system of medicine than Charles Reade, who, in one of his works, gives the opinion of Dr. Sampson, a character original for the period, who was evidently opposed to the antiphlogistic method of treatment, and who contended that he could tell, beforehand, every prescription which would be given by the different prominent physicians of his time. In his conversation with a patient, who had been consulting the most celebrated physicians she could reach, he says: "Good heavens! madam, what a gauntlet of gabies for a woman to run and come out alive. These four physicians you have been to see are specialists, that means—monomaniacs. They have advised the antiphlogistic regimen, have they? Antiphlogistic, my dear madam, that one long fragment of asses jaw has slain a million. The antophlogistic theory is this, that disease is fiery, and that any exhaustion of the vital force must cool the system and reduce the morbid fire, called, in their donkey latin, flamma, and in their compound donkey latin, inflammation; and, accordingly, the antiphlogistic practice is to cool the sick man by bleeding him, and when bled, either to re-bleed him with a change of instrument—bites and stabs, instead of gashes or blisters, and push mercury till the teeth of the bled man rake and shake in their sockets, and to salivate from first to last. As for blood-letting, it is inflammatory, for the thumping heart and bounding pulse of patients, bled by butchers in black, and bullocks bled by butchers in blue, prove it.

I wonder they didn't inventory satan and his brimstone lake among their refrigerators."

"What is the cause of that rare event which occurs only to patients who can't afford doctoring, death from old age? His bodily expenses go on. His bodily income falls off, by failure of the reparative and reproductive forces."

"Whatever the disease, its form and essence, expenditure goes on and income lessens." But to the sick, and therefore weak man, comes a doctor, who pronounces him an invalid, gashes him with a lancet, spills out the great liquid material of all repair by the gallon, and fells this weak man, wounded now, pale and fainting, with death stamped on his face, to the earth like a bayoneted soldier or a slaughtered ox.

If the weak man, wounded thus and weakened, survives, then the chartered thugs, who have drained him by the bung hole, turned to and drain him by the spigot.

They blister him and then calomel him, and lest nature should have the ghost of a chance to counterbalance these frightful out-goings, they keep strong meat and drink out of his system, emptied by their stabs, bites, purges, mercury and blisters.

Antiphlogistic is but a modern name for ass—assinating, which has never varied a hair since scholastic medicine. The silliest and deadliest of all the hundred forms of quackery first rose—unlike science, art, religion, and all true suns in the west, to wound the sick, to weaken the weak, to mutilate the hurt, and thin mankind."

This was the method of treatment adopted by the old school

physicians in Pittsburgh at the time your pioneer, Dr. Reichhelm, crossed yonder range of mountains to establish a rational method of treatment in your city. Since that time, how things have changed!

The lancet has been discarded, mercury has been laid upon the shelf, emetics and violent cathartics have been thrown to the dogs. What has worked this wonderful change?

It is conceded by prominent old school authors that it was from the Homœopaths that they learned that all this barbarous, murderous treatment was unnecessary.

Niemeyer said, on examining the bodies of persons dying of pneumonia treated according to the method formerly so universal: "We find so very little blood in the heart and arteries that we are tempted to ascribe death to the treatment rather than the disease."

Yes, old school medicine has undergone a change,—a decided change, and for the better. But this, from the *Medical Record* of September 3d, of this year, the old school journal having the largest circulation of any medical journal in the United States, proves that with all this modification it has not as yet diminished its death rate to that of the Homœopathic school. I quote from the journal named:

"The annual reports of the Cook County Hospital (located in Chicago) reveal some facts in which the profession should feel some interest. On the opening pages we find a list of the members of the regular medical board, and below of the Homœopathic medical board. Such juxtaposition seems a little at variance with conventional ethics, but in this we may be mistaken.

"The point that is of real importance, is that both in its totals and in the medical and surgical departments, the mortality of patients treated by the Homœopathic medical board is less than that of the regular medical board, and this is true, not for one year, but apparently for a series of years."

This statement alone, appearing, as it does, in the leading old school medical journal of America, speaks volumes for the advances which homœopathy has made in the United States.

Formerly it was persecution, ridicule, participated in by the people, too. *Just fifty years* ago our method of treatment was first introduced in the city of Pittsburgh. In that comparatively short time the eyes of the people have been opened, and they have learned that disease can be cured without resorting to the nauseous doses, the tortures and depletion considered necessary then to save life, and, as a result, instead of having one solitary physician west of the Alleghenies practicing according to the homœopathic law of cure, they can be numbered by the thousand; well educated, too, both as physicians and surgeons, whose patrons are among the best educated and most prominent of our citizens.

Not long since a leading New York physician said to me "Doctor, you homœopathists have entirely too large a share of the wealth and intellect of New York among your patrons. The fact is, doctor, an ignorant man cannot realize that he is deriving any benefit from medicine unless he sees its effect; he must be purged, vomited, blistered or bled, or he thinks nothing is being done. These patients we retain."

How common it was in old times to hear a patient say, "I did not send for you, doctor, because I could not afford to be sick." It was the rule, and they knew it, for a patient to be made worse before he recovered from his malady.

But all this has been done away with, never again to be revived. The success of our school, and all here are familiar with it, has far surpassed the expectations of our honored pioneers. Scarcely a city, town or village in the United States where homœopathy is not successfully practiced; and so it is throughout the civilized world.

They say the two schools are converging. I trust ours will remain a straight line,—the other will reach us and unite in time. Angry dispute will be done away with, and it will be conceded that honest convictions should be respected.

No discord will arise to mar our labors, for our calling is a noble one. In the language of a distinguished medical orator, "Our profession is inferior to none, as noble an art as any that taxes the intellect of man. At all times, in all seasons, under every variety of circumstances are our ministrations sought; the summer's heat and winter's cold, storm and sunshine, night and day alike witness our labors and attest our fidelity. Among the vehicles which throng your city's crowded streets at mid-day you may mark the roll of the physician's wheels; and in the still, small hours of night you may hear the sound of his footstep as he traverses the deserted pavements on some errand of mercy. The navy! Is there a blood-stained deck on which he is not found? The army! Is there a battle-field without him? Nay, is he not often the last to leave the scene of slaughter, remaining a voluntary prisoner to the enemy, whose persevering columns find him at his post, ministering to friend and foe alike. The pulpit! Our duties to the human race begin with the first feeble breath of the new born infant, and we are the watchful sentries to the building until its due expansion shall enable it to receive those treasures with which the minister is prepared to store it. Henceforth our duties lie side by side; body and soul within our united keeping until a greater and mightier minister than either shall dismiss the guard."

I have detained you longer than I ought, but I will have traveled nearly a thousand miles to be with you to-day. I will now close, and with your permission will continue with the consideration of the progress of homœopathic medicine at your centennial celebration—fifty years from this day.

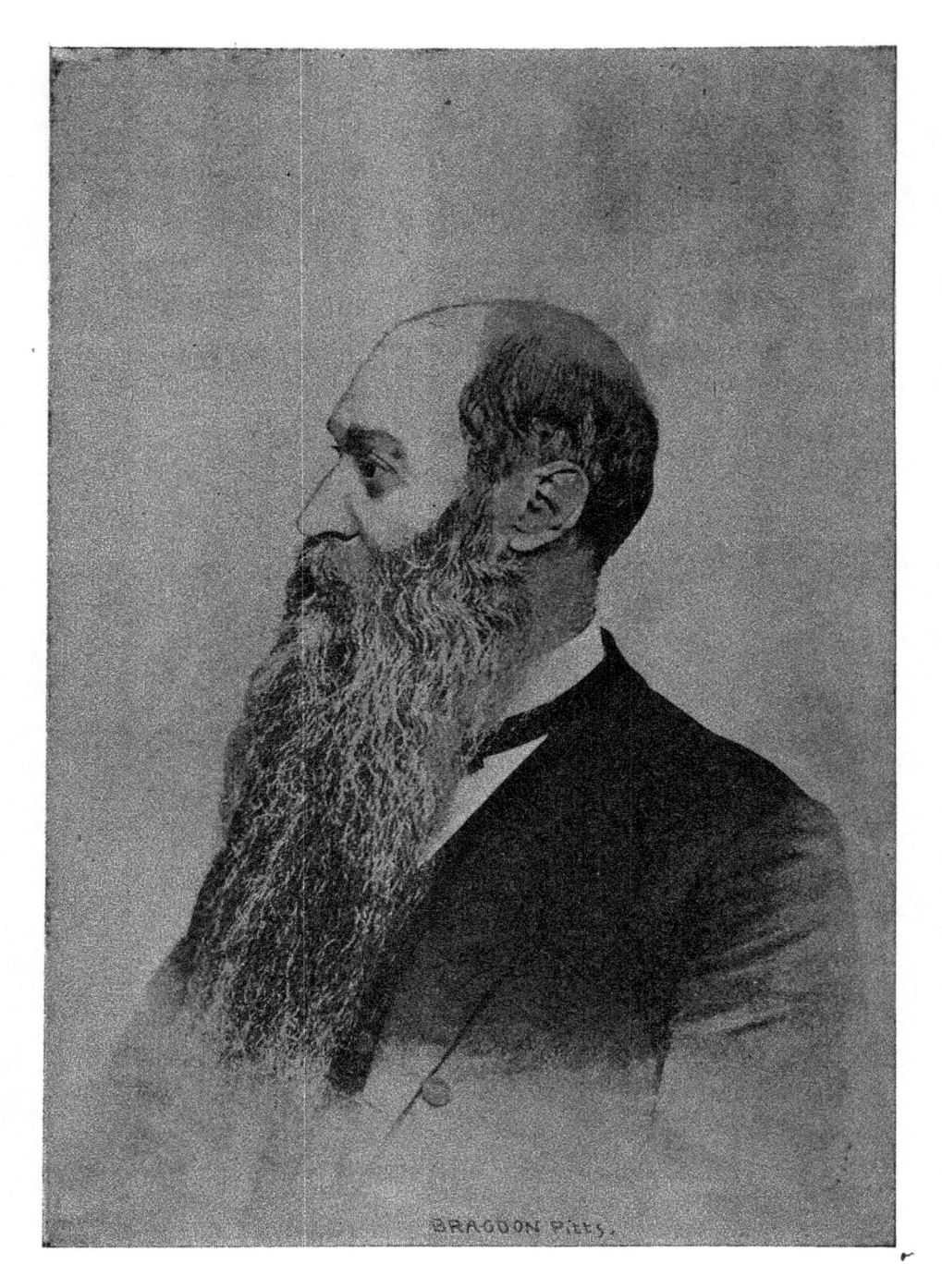

J. C. Burgher

ADDRESS,

By J. C. Burgher, M.D., of Pittsburgh, Pa.

Mr. Chairman, Ladies and Gentlemen:

As President of the Homœopathic Medical Society of Allegheny County, under whose patronage this celebration is held, I have been called upon to say something in commemoration of the event. The honor accorded to me to offer a tribute commemorative of the pioneers of Homœopathy West of the Alleghenies, I most thankfully accept and cheerfully embrace. And yet, it places me in a position peculiarly embarrassing, from the fact that my eloquent and distinguished confréres who have preceded me have anticipated my speech. They seem to have made a division among themselves of what I had intended to say and "cast lots" for it. The best, therefore, that I can possibly do will be to *re-vamp* it and offer it as second-hand matter.

The successful introduction of Homœopathy in this city, fifty years ago, by its able, accomplished and conscientious champion, Gustavus Reichhelm, M.D., marks an epoch in the history of medicine, the most remarkable in the records of time. Remarkable alike for the persistent opposition, prejudice, ridicule and misstatements with which it had to contend and the triumphs it has achieved.

Fifty years ago the practice of medicine was a monopoly that exerted all its power and influence to repel and crush everything new in the "healing art;" to reject, without trial or investigation, every innovation from that which was taught in the schools of the day. Fifty years ago the medical profession constituted a close corporation that made every effort in its power to confine the practice of medicine to its individual members, who persistently adhered to that practice in its stereotyped and orthodox form. With these indisputable facts before us, need we wonder that Dr. Reichhelm was denounced by his Allopathic contemporaries as a charlatan and humbug, ostracised by the clergy, boycotted by the druggists, and looked upon with suspicion by the community? Dr. Reichhelm's natural ability was above that of the average physician of his time; his scholastic attainments were broad and comprehensive, and his degree in medicine was conferred by one of the leading universities of his day. And yet he did not, in his own estimation, know too much to search for more light and investigate anything that gave promise of more satisfactory results. After a long and critical investigation of Homœopathy under the guidance of Drs. Hering, Wesselhœft, Detwiler and other members of the faculty of the Allentown Academy of Medicine, he was firmly convinced of its superiority in the treatment of disease, and had the courage to discard the practice and teachings of Allopathy and the boldness to dispute the sovereignty of antimony, opium, calomel and jalap, as well as their Ajax Telemon and ubiquitous accomplice, the lancet. He came here as an exponent of a new science and art of healing, based upon an immutable *law*. Its methods and teachings were utterly at variance with everything at that *time* considered orthodox in medicine. He came here with the firm conviction of the truth and ultimate triumph of the Heaven-ordained law of cure that guided him in his practice. He came here to *stay*, and he introduced Homœopathy here to abide as an enduring legacy to the sick and suffering until *time* shall have been succeeded by *eternity*.

From this small beginning how rapid the progress and immense the extension of the therapeutic principles introduced here by Dr. Reichhelm, within the memory of many present to-day!

Some of the noble fruits of the extension of Homœopathy are, that it has taken the old school with it, so far as to very greatly modify and improve its teachings and practice by forcing it to abandon the lancet, and to substitute small doses for the large ones formerly prescribed. It has emancipated the minds of the practitioners of the dominant school of to-day from the degrading bondage of many long-cherished errors and deeply-rooted prejudices of their predecessors; while the intolerance, discourtesy, ridicule and contempt to which the disciples of Hahnemann were treated by their Allopathic contemporaries have rapidly passed into inglorious desuetude. While the auxiliary sciences, Anatomy, Physiology, Biology, Pathology, Surgery, etc., have kept pace with other branches of scientific knowledge the past half century, the *materia medica* and therapeutics of the dominant school, by its own admission, are as empirical and uncertain now as they were in the past.

The International Medical Congress, (to which Dr. Dowling has referred), met in Washington, D. C., the second week of this present month, and continued in session for several days. Its delegates were composed of the most eminent physicians from every civilized nation on the earth. The transactions of this great international gathering of learned physicians furnish us with the results of many interesting experiments and discoveries, of more or less practical value in the various collateral sciences of medicine, while the present state of medicine proper (*materia medica* and *therapeutics*), was submitted in an essay read before the section of *therapeutics*, Sept. 8th, 1887, by Dr. Samuel S. Wallian, in which he says: "The contradictory and opposite qualities and powers ascribed to drugs used as remedies are a constant stumbling block to students of medicine. The properties ascribed to many of them to-day are opposite of those with which the same substances stood accredited twenty years ago. The old *cardiac depressants* are now *cardiac 'tonics,'* and *vice versa.* All this proves their unreliability. To the thoughtful reasoner it suggests, if it does not prove, far more; and that is that the whole theory of their alleged '*action*' is based on questionable premises."

This is an honest confession of the empiricism of the Allopathic school of medicine at the present time, by one occupying a prominent position in the profession. This is the inevitable result of any therapeutic method based on a *materia medica* made up of empirical knowledge, limited to a narrow range of loose and inexact observations.

In 1842 Dr. C. Bayer located in Allegheny City, and in 1846 Dr. D. M. Dake settled in this city; soon after Drs. M. Côté, H. H. Hofmann, Wm. Penniman and F. Taudte, all educated in old school medicine, located here as Homœopathic physicians, followed by Drs. J. F. Cooper, J. P. Dake and others present with us to-day. At this date there are over seventy Homœopathic physicians in active practice in Allegheny county. Fifty years ago there was but one West of the Allegheny mountains. Now there are more than five thousand. Fifty years ago there was not a single book on the principles and practice of Homœopathy in the English language; now the medical literature of Homœopathy in the English language alone constitutes a large medical library. Fifty years ago there was not a single medical journal published in the interest of Homœopathy; now there are twenty-eight in the United States regularly issued and liberally patronized. When Dr. Reichhelm introduced Homœopathy as a new and better method of healing than any that had preceded it, there was not a Homœopathic medical college in the world; now there are thirteen in the United States, whose facilities for medical instruction in all its branches are not excelled by any medical college in the country, and are equaled by very few, if any. Fifty years ago there was not a Homœopathic hospital, dispensary, or medical society in the world; now there are fifty-seven Homœopathic hospitals in this country alone, three insane asylums, forty-eight public dispensaries, one hundred and fifty medical societies, and over ten thousand Homœopathic physicians The past year has furnished more accessions to the professional ranks of Homœopathy than in any other equal period of time in its important and eventful history.

> If this be the lustre of its dawning name,
> Who can paint it in its noonday fame?

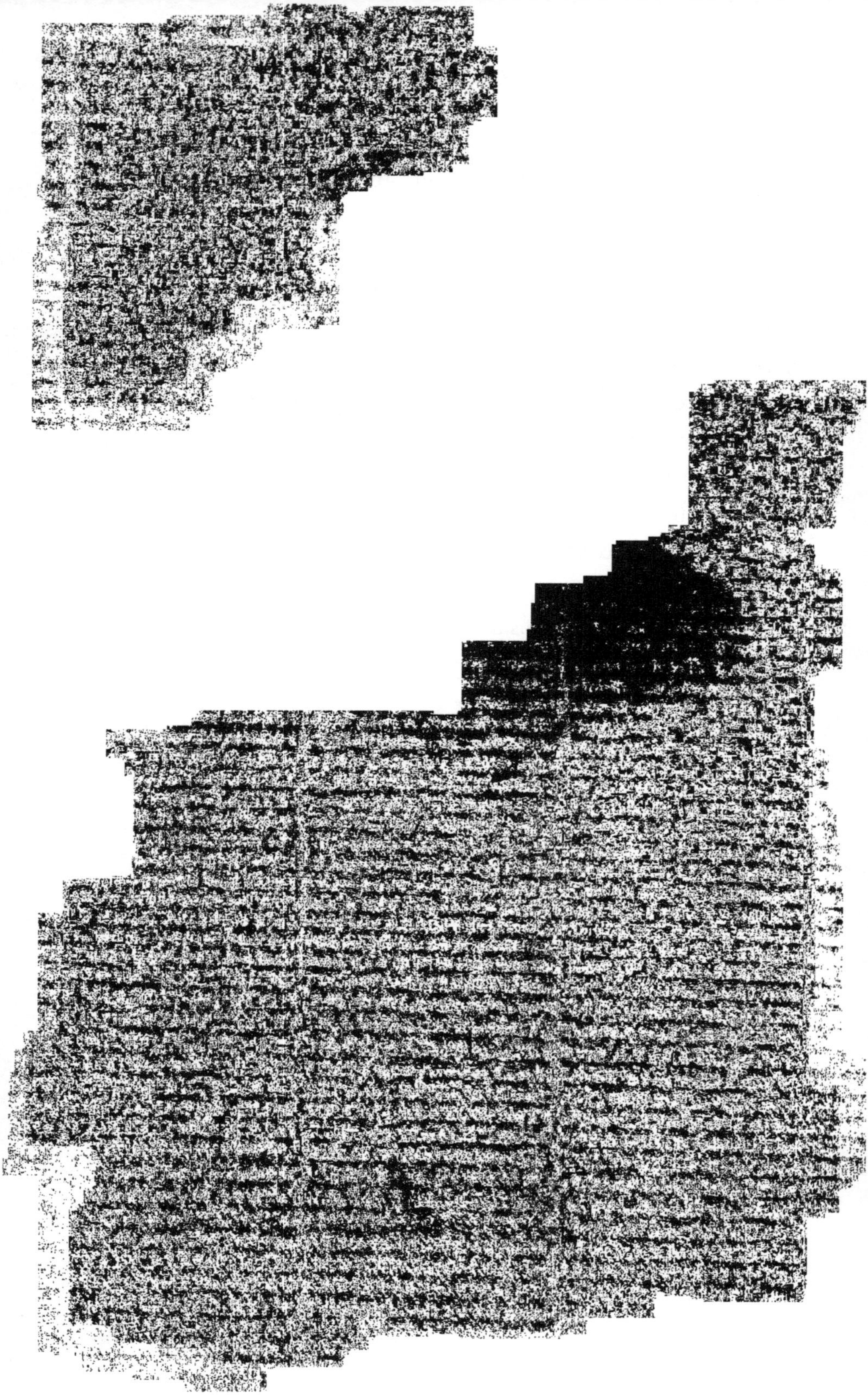

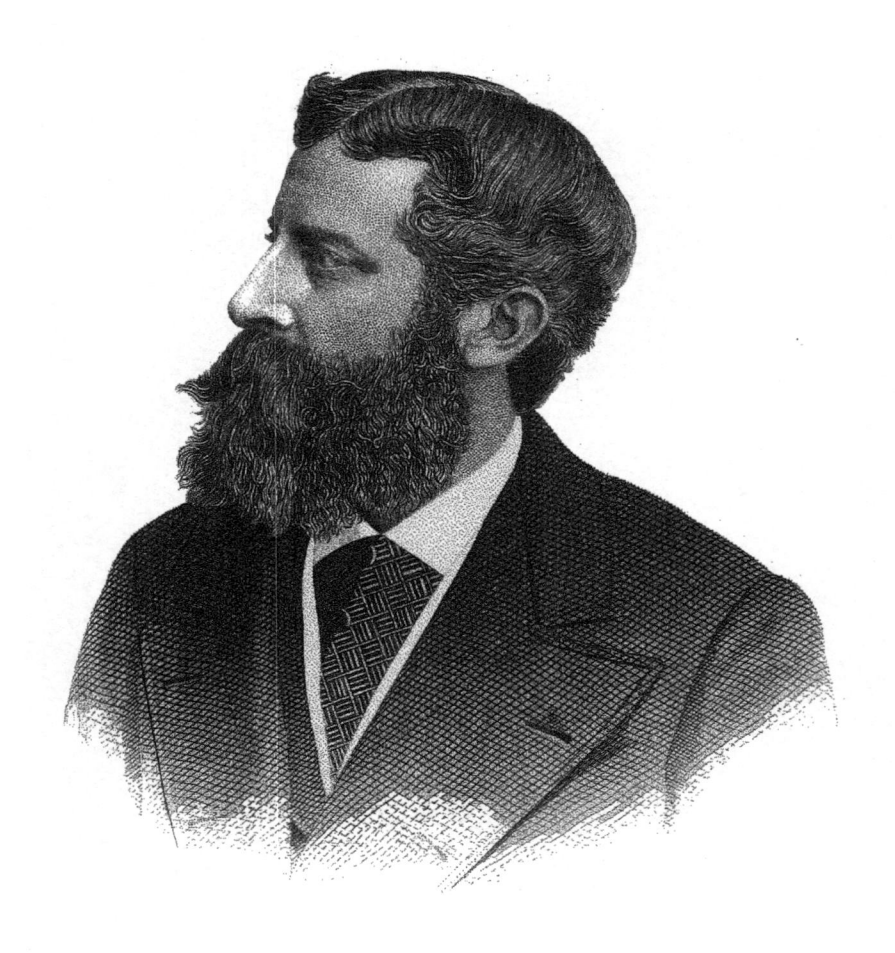

Eng⁴ by Geo E Perine, N York

DOGMATIC DOCTORS.

A SATIRE.

By Wm. Tod Helmuth, M.D., New York, N. Y.

The great Apollo, radiant and strong,
Was God of Physic, e'en while God of Song,
Disdaining neither mortar nor scalpel,
While from his lyre impassioned love strains fell.
So may a Doctor, humble though he be,
Aspire awhile to flights of minstrelsy;
Forget his powders and his pills discard;
Become at once a medicated bard,
Whose numbers, flowing smoothly as they will,
Exhale both Nux and Belladonna still.
The winged horse sprang from Medusa's blood,
Which well'd from wounds by Perseus made a flood;
Therefore a Surgeon, by this right divine,
May deal with dactyls in heroic line,
And, whispering up the glades of Phocis, may
Ask aid for his hexameters to-day.
And if the Muse in one short hour should tell
Of occult truths, professional, which dwell
Within the sacred precincts of the craft,
Restrain your judgment;—think the poet daft.

Doctors resemble very jealous lovers,
One sneers at that the other one discovers;
One may declare that he the truth descries,
The other flatly tells you that he lies.
The one announces that a new bacillus

Will breed a pestilence and surely kill us;
The other, laughing, says this mundane sphere,
Minus the microbe, soon would disappear.
One swears malaria will ever be
The fountain head of each infirmity;
The other proves diseases to be fewer,
'Mongst those who daily labor in the sewer.
And so dogmatic doctors dodge the blow
Which brother doctors on their heads bestow.

So when a principle, which, if believed,
Would overturn all notions preconceived,
Would sadly sully Æsculapian fame,
And cast discredit on " old Physics' " name,
Came like the spark, which little power displays,
Till winds propitious fan it to blaze—
The doctors, still dogmatic, rose *en masse*,
Called the progenitor of truth an ass;
Sneer'd at his knowledge, and his name reviled,
Sland'rous reproach on misconstruction piled,
Bound him at once on persecution's rack,
Term'd nature's greatest benefactor, " Quack; "
Lampooned the scholar with a ribald wit,
With arguments at once unjust, unfit;
Including, in their universal ban,
The life, the works, the friends of Hahnemann.

When Pyrrhus, so the ancient fable goes,
Was eager marching on Bercean foes,
A spirit from immortal Mars was sent
To summon him to Alexander's tent.
There, spent with wounds, the Macedonian lay,
But promised succor in the coming fray.
" How can this be? " th' indignant Pyrrhus cries,
" The light of life is failing in thine eyes,
Thy marshal spirit can inspire no more,
To-morrow thou shalt touch the Stygian shore."

The mighty chieftain raised his mailed hand,
And thus to Pyrrhus, in most stern command:
" Yet shalt thou triumph both by land and sea,
Still shall thy gonfalon victorious be,
Still shall the pæan echo with thy fame,
For I will lead thine armies by my name."
And so the name of Hahnemann shall be
The watch-word for diseased humanity,
When that vast army of the body's foes,
Of aches and pains and agonies composed,
That ever watchful in our earthly span
Descend rapaciously on erring man,
Obstruct his life-work with their baleful breath,
Ofttimes the *avant couriers* of death.

Yet spite of all reproach the system grew,
Extending from the old world to the new;
Sweeping away objections in its flight,
Gathering, in its momentum, might;
Each fact established tending to create
An increased spirit to investigate.
Then Gram and Hering from the master came,
And still, like Pyrrhus, trusting in a name,
With faith implicit in the cause did rear
Its banner on the Western Hemisphere.
Here was the soil in which to plant the seed,
Here toleration greeted every creed,
Here new philosophy new truths displayed,
And day by day were new discoveries made.
Here the profession liberal would be
And gladly welcome homœopathy.
Vain was the surmise and the hope forlorn,
The doctors, still dogmatic, laughed in scorn,
Smelt at their canes and prophesying swore
In half a decade 't would be known no more.
" What," cried these dignified and learned M.D.'s,
" If like cures like, disease must cure disease.

This is paradox, a child may see,
To all established teaching contrary.
The Æsculapian temple stands disgraced
Till this unfounded tenet is displaced,
No mortal since Hippocrates was born,
Save Paracelsus, drunken and forlorn,
Has dared our precincts sacred to invade,
And shake foundations centuries have laid.
Make Mother Goose the text book of this school,
In rhymes she tells the children of a fool,
Whose eyes scratched out, with all his might and main
With sharper briars scratched them in again."

So against the master and his law of cure,
His name reviled, his system's downfall sure,
The critics judgment gave, in language gross,
But grew more rabid when they came to dose.
" Put but a drop of aconite," say they,
" In winter months on rocks in Baffin's Bay,
In spring-tide let the homœopathist go
Rejoicing to the Gulf of Mexico,
Drop there a vial in the waves so bright,
And draw from thence the potent aconite.
Immediate cork it, shake the bottle well,
Give fever'd patients every hour a smell,
And see disease, ere that olfaction's done,
Vanish like mist before the morning sun."
Thus ridicule its sharpest arrow sent
As substitute for solid argument.
But ridicule can offer slight defense
'Gainst facts established by our common sense.

As yet, beyond the Alleghenies blue,
Adherents to the system were but few,
Till sent by Hering, Gustave Reichhelm came,
Like Gram and Pyrrhus, trusting in a name.
Remember this was fifty years ago,

Travel to westward then was wondrous slow,
No rushing trains by hundreds every day
Like light'ning speeded over the iron way,
No tunneled mountains echoed with the scream
Of iron horses with their breath of steam;
No velvet-cushioned, ventilated car;
No Pullman patent trains vestibular;
To rails of steel, no Westinghouse's brake,
Which now the journey so luxurious make,
Were known to man. Conveyance then was rude,
The journey hither one of magnitude;
The cumbrous stage coach climb'd the steep ascent,
While dang'rous passes to the journey lent
Increasing peril to the traveler, who
By force of circumstance came through.
Yet all undaunted came the pioneer
To Pittsburgh, then considered a frontier.
Alone, this solitary German youth,
Simple in mind, relying on the truth,
Without a partisan, without a friend
On whom in times of trial to depend,
Unknown but patient, steadfast and sincere,
Unfurled his banner, which he planted here.
Behold! what half a century has done;
To-day we thank him for the battle won.
Friends, can you dream how fast the pulses be
Of this great age, the last half century?

Add skill to force and see ten thousand powers
Shake the great earth in these fast times of ours;
See, in five decades what our race has done,
Grand in the past, but grander yet to come.
Thousands of slaves from galling chains set free,
And man of man demanding liberty.
Of speech, of action and of wholesome thought,
Which widening science in our times has wrought,
Behold where woman, better understood,

Stands in the glory of her womanhood,
Freed from that prejudice, where long confined,
Her body was acknowledged, not her mind;
See where the microscope has opened wide
The gates of science where we petrified;
Behold new fields, revealing though untrod,
The increased wisdom of Almighty God.

But here in Pittsburgh, fifty years ago,
These mighty changes had not stirred men so.
The horizon, 'tis true, was fair and bright,
Glowing and beautiful with coming light,
But doctors, still dogmatic in their pride,
Though waking slowly to the rising tide
Of views enlarging and of newer thought,
Still held the doctrines that their fathers taught,
Mistrusted every innovation bold,
Despised the new, but reverenced the old.
These were the times when, daily, " ten and ten "
Relieved the livers of our fellow men,
When blisters set the epidermis free,
When stabbing pains foretold a pleurisy;
When blood in streamlets was allowed to run
In every case there was a doubt upon;
When seton's, moxa's and the issue peas,
Combined or singly frightened off disease,
Which often with rapidity withdrew,
Relieved the pain, but killed the patient too.

Then, as before to Gram—now Reichhelm's foes,
Dogmatic Doctors instantly arose,
Who like their brothers, centuries before
Great Harvey villified, at Jenner swore,
In old examples satisfaction found,
And made with ridicule the air resound,
" Humbug! most arrant humbug!" was the cry;
" Give it a decade and the thing will die."
Thus did dogmatic doctors prophesy.

Men rent with pain care not for science,
'Tis then the doctor is their chief reliance.
Migrating microbes are forgot in spasm,
And all the varied forms of bioplasm
Drop from the convolutions of the brain
E'en of the scientist when racked with pain.
That man who quickest cures them of their ills,
Reducing to a minimum their bills,
With nauseating drugs disgusts them least,
Of Æsculapius is the true high priest.
To him successful—sure as shines the sun—
Afflicted mortals will determined run,
One cure effected here produced another,
Each man made whole informed his suf'ring brother
That a new system, how, he could not tell,
But minus opium or calomel,
Had cured his ills, his biting pangs relieved,
That cures were facts and must be believed.
So with a force unknown by Heaven blest,
The system of spreading fill'd the distant west.
When Reichhelm came, now fifty years ago,
Pittsburgh herself could scarce her future know.
Behold her now, her forces still unspent,
The greatest factor on this continent.
See, where her hills the untold iron hold,
Which rules the world more certainly than gold;
See, in her mines the everlasting coal;
Here in her streets the hum, the whirr, the roll,
A million wheels develop and command
The skill'd attention of the workman's hand.
Nature's great forces now are said to be
Pure light, great heat and electricity.
Pittsburghians have caught and chain'd the three,
Made them obedient to inventive will,
While untold wonders are predicted still.

What heat for regulation can surpass
Caloric furnished by your natural gas?
Where is illumination half so bright
As here where shines the incandescent light
Which through a wire-electric instant flies?
A touch ignites it—by a touch it dies.
Here flames the furnace, there the forge by night
Reddens the firmament with lurid light.
And yonder factories, 'mid fire and smoke,
Produce ten hundred thousand tons of coke
In one short year; and see the adjacent soil
Yielding in torrents lubricating oil;
While clanging hammers and anvils' ring
Proudly proclaim your "iron city"—King.

As progress opens wide these new domains
Fair science liberality proclaims.
Physicians, once material, can show
That great results from smallest forces grow;
That all the atmosphere is filled with germs,
Arranged and classified with curious terms;
That each disease a special microbe claims
With scientific though jaw-breaking names,
That in our food, our ice, the air, the ground,
Bacteria subtle everywhere abound.
That life itself, with all its joys and woes,
Comes from a bioplast which no one knows.
They call it protoplasmic, and it grows.
The microscopists of to-day can tell
That man himself is nothing but a *sell*.

With these o'erwhelming revelations known,
The doctors now have less dogmatic grown,
Each honest man—*but honest he must be*—
Allows his friends the utmost liberty
To cure his sick, as conscience may direct,
Without regard to "pathy" or to sect,

For old-time dogmatism now forsooth
Is overpower'd by the march of truth.
For truth is golden, beautiful and pure,
Though error ofttimes may its path obscure;
The voice of rancor may its progress mar,
As sombre clouds eclipse the brightest star;
Ancient opinions may obstruct its light,
And misconception veil it from our sight—
Yet as the mists of old delusions fade,
And fierce invective sinks into the shade,
Truth's glorious light will then refulgent shine
Undimmed and peerless by a right divine;
For God is truth, and truth must ever be
In man a near approach to Deity.

WESTWARD THE STAR SIMILIA TAKES ITS WAY.

By T. P. Wilson, M.D., Ann Arbor, Mich.

O'er lofty Alleghenies, forest crowned,
   Through untold ages swept the mighty sun;
And eagles from their towering æries found
   No path of human progress yet begun.

Now, at their teeming bases cities rise,
   And fruitful fields o'erspread their glowing sides;
And millions look with proud and happy eyes
   Where Peace with Plenty regal power divides.

Lo! from the East, the glowing light we see,
   Where brightly gleams Similia's rising star.
Before its coming, Death and Darkness flee,
   And Hope's bright gates of gold are left ajar.

Though but a half a century ago,
   It leaped the mountain's bold and rugged crest,
It lighteth every path that man may go,
   And flecks with glory all the broad'ning West.

To Hahnemann and Reichhelm well we give
   All honor, which to them is just and due;
Immortal in our praise they ever live,
   Because, to thee, O! loved *Similia*, true.

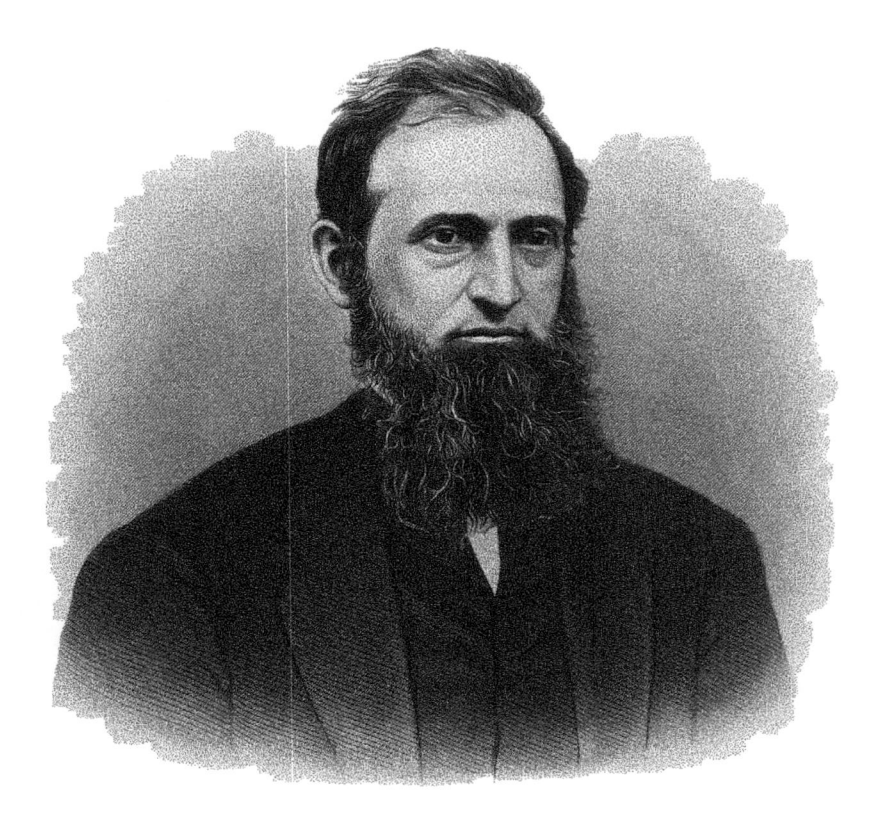

Galaxy Pub. Co Philada

J. F. Cooper

List of Officers and Members
—of—
THE HOMŒOPATHIC MEDICAL SOCIETY
—of—
ALLEGHENY COUNTY, PENNSYLVANIA.

OFFICERS.

1887.

President,	J. C. Burgher, M.D.
Vice-President,	J. F. Cooper, M.D.
Secretary,	C. H. Hofmann, M.D.
Treasurer,	J. B. McClelland, M.D.

Censors:

C. C. Rinehart, M.D.   L. H. Willard, M.D

J. H. McClelland, M.D.

Executive Committee:

J. F. Cooper, M.D.,   L. H. Willard, M..D.,

Wm. R. Childs, M.D.,   W. H. Winslow, M.D.

J. H. McClelland, M.D.

1888.

President,	J. F. Cooper, M.D.
Vice-President,	Z. T. Miller, M.D.
Secretary,	J. Richey Horner, M.D.
Treasurer,	J. B. McClelland, M.D.

Censors:

C. C. Rinehart, M.D.,   L. H. Willard, M.D.,

J. H. McClelland, M.D.

Executive Committee:

J. C. BURGHER, M.D.,   J. H. MCCLELLAND, M.D.,
WM. R. CHILDS, M.D.,   L. H. WILLARD, M.D.,
W. H. WINSLOW, M.D.

Members:

C. F. BINGAMAN, M.D.
M. C. BLYSTONE, M.D.
E. E. BRIGGS, M.D.
J. C. BURGHER, M.D.
M. J. CHAPMAN, M.D.
I. B. CHANTLER, M.D.
WM. R. CHILDS, M.D.
J. F. COOPER, M.D.
JOHN COOPER, M.D.
MARGARET L. CRUMPTON, M.D.
S. W. S. DINSMORE, M.D.
W. F. EDMUNDSON, M.D.
R. K. FLEMING, M.D.
JOHN L. FERSON, M.D.
H. W. FULTON, M.D.
CHAS. GANGLOFF, M.D.
F. H. GRIMES, M.D.
F. C. GUNDLACH, M D.
C. D. HERRON, M.D.
C. H. HOFMANN, M.D.
H. H. HOFMANN, M.D.
J. RICHEY HORNER, M.D
W. H. KERN, M.D.
WM. D. KING, M.D.
W. J. MARTIN, M.D.

J. B. MCCLELLAND, M.D.
J. H. MCCLELLAND, M.D.
R. W. MCCLELLAND, M.D.
T. T. MCNISH, M.D.
Z T. MILLER, M.D.
G. A. MUELLER, M.D.
R. V. PITCAIRN, M.D.
R. Y. RAMAGE, M.D.
J. S. RANKIN, M.D.
W. C. RANSON, M.D.
C. C. RINEHART, M.D.
J. F. ROBERTS, M.D.
L G. ROUSSEAU, M.D.
C. P. SEIP, M.D.
O. R. SHANNON, M.D.
S. F. SHANNON, M.D.
MARY E. SMITH, M.D.
PEARL STARR, M.D.
J. BAILEY SULLIVAN, M.D.
J. H. THOMPSON, M.D.
F. P. WILCOX, M.D.
L. H. WILLARD, M.D.
CHAS. A. WILSON, M.D.
W. H. WINSLOW, M.D.
W. W. WOLFE, M.D.